T0279617

# STRESS AND INFLAMMATION

# STRESS AND INFLAMMATION

## A Silent Epidemic

Larry Davis, DC
Lenae White, MD

BROWN BOOKS
PUBLISHING GROUP

*Stress and Inflammation*
*A Silent Epidemic*

Brown Books Publishing Group
Dallas, TX / New York, NY
www.BrownBooks.com
(972) 381-0009

A New Era in Publishing®

Publisher's Cataloging-in-Publication
Names: Davis, Larry, 1962- author. | White, Lenae, author.
Title: Stress and inflammation : a silent epidemic / Larry Davis, DC [and] Lenae White, MD.
Description: Dallas, TX ; New York, NY : Brown Books Publishing Group, [2022] | Includes
    bibliographical references.
Identifiers: ISBN: 9781612545509 (hardcover) | LCCN: 2021921877
Subjects: LCSH: Stress (Physiology)--Health aspects. | Inflammation—Alternative treatment.
    | Stress (Physiology)--Nutritional aspects. | Stress management. | Nutrition. | Health
    behavior. | BISAC: HEALTH & FITNESS / Diet & Nutrition / General. | SELF-HELP /
    Self-Management / Stress Management.
Classification: LCC: RA785 .D38 2022 | DDC: 616.9/8--dc23

ISBN 978-1-61254-550-9
LCCN 2021921877

Printed in the United States
10 9 8 7 6 5 4 3 2 1

For more information or to contact the author, please go to
www.VitalityEP.com.

*I would like to dedicate this book to my life partner, Faye Spiegel, RN,
who has supported me through my research and holistic practice
for the past twenty years.*
*—Larry Davis*


*To my mom and dad:*
*Mom, you went to heaven way too soon. You are my inspiration for
pursuing the information presented in this book. Thank you for
all that you did to make everyone's life better, especially mine!
This is for you—I love you, Mom, and I miss you every day!*

*Dad, you worked long hours to help make all my dreams possible;
you are my inspiration for pushing through to the end—thank you.
You never stopped loving me and believing in me.
This is for you—I love you, Dad!*
*—Lenae White*

# Table of Contents

## Part III: The Plan

## Conclusion

## Appendices

## Notes

## Illustration Credits

## About the Authors

# Preface

This book is a result of the combined fifty years of work with patients in clinical practice for Dr. Larry Davis, DC, and Dr. Lenae White, MD. The information in this book is the culmination of a wide variety of clinical experiences in lifestyle medicine. The authors have worked together on this book to give you some of the same information they have found to be life-changing and re-energizing. Their hope is that you are able to use this information to heal, to replenish, and to restore the energy you once had as a child.

Although Dr. Davis has a doctorate degree in chiropractics and a fellowship in acupuncture, just a few years into his chiropractic practice, he found himself turning to clinical physiology when faced with a serious health crisis involving his thyroid gland. After successfully resolving this thyroid condition using holistic treatment, he focused all of his post-graduate education on endocrinology (the study of hormones). For the last twenty years, he has worked with thousands of people, helping them to achieve optimal wellness by natural means, through nutrition, supplementation, exercise, developing optimal sleep habits, and meditation.

Dr. White has twenty-five years in clinical practice. She earned her MD degree, completed four years of internship/residency at MAYO Clinic, and completed a three-year addiction fellowship at the University of Pennsylvania. Although she has a doctorate in allopathic medicine, she, too, turned to clinical physiology and lifestyle medicine to address significant health issues that developed from a severe adrenal gland dysfunction. After successfully resolving her issues, she has since been focusing on incorporating optimal wellness and creating long-lasting lifestyle changes for her patients.

# Acknowledgments

We would like to acknowledge and thank all the researchers, doctors, and health practitioners who have inspired us, specifically Dr. Ray Peat, PhD and Georgi Dinkov, MSc for their extensive writings and lectures on physiology and biochemistry, which have helped solidify our views on health. We also would like to acknowledge the pioneers of the bioenergetic model of health such as Gilbert Ling, PhD, Albert Szent-Györgyi, MD, PhD, Hans Selye, MD, PhD, Dr. Broda Barnes, MD, and many other great minds who challenged the medical model and traditional thinking.

We want to especially thank Brown Books Publishing for selecting our manuscript, for all of their hard work, and for the many hours they spent with us helping us through every step of the publishing process. We are very grateful to have this opportunity to start a conversation with America on battling the chronic stress we are all living with on a daily basis. We want to say a special thanks to our editors, graphic design team, and all those who committed their time, talent, and expertise to our book. And a very special thanks to Tom Reale, president/COO, for believing in us and providing us a platform to get this information out.

# Introduction

The life-destroying effects of stress and inflammation can be seen in nearly everyone in our society. In our modern society, no one is absent or immune to stress.

It doesn't matter whether you are a construction worker or the CEO of a large company—we all have stress. We are living in a time of unprecedented and ongoing chronic stressors. Stress can come in the form of financial hardships, relationships, family, health, natural disasters, and the list goes on and on.

We have seen in clinical practice that stress, and especially ongoing chronic stress, can have a devastating effect on our lives and can present with many different symptoms. For one person, it may start as anxiety/depression, it may be fatigue for someone else, and for another it can be hormonal dysfunction. There are many people who never realize that stress may be the underlying cause of an autoimmune disease and/or chronic health condition(s). What is clear in the research is that stress and inflammation play a role in almost all chronic health conditions. Though science tries to look for the gene that is causing the problem and the next gene therapy to cure the problem, it usually comes back to stress, inflammation, and an overall lowered physical energy state. The more energy the body has, and the more balanced our hormones are, the better we can deal with the assault of stress, inflammation, pathogens, and any other health issues that may arise.

Why do we need another book on health and wellness when there are thousands of books already written?

This book is unlike any book before. In these pages, you will not find what conventional medicine and the mainstream media will tell you. If they had the answers, we would not have the health problems that we do. We would not worry about protecting the people with comorbidities (pre-existing conditions) from COVID-19. We would not have cancer, heart disease, and medicine as the top three causes of death every year.

It is not that the current medical model is wrong; it just looks at the body as a collection of parts that act independently from each other, as if it is a car or other type of machine. How else can you explain every type of specialist in the medical field? The cardiologist looks at the heart and prescribes medication to lower blood pressure, not always identifying the cause of the problem. The oncologist tries to rid the body of cancer, not always pursuing or addressing the underlying cause(s) of the cancer like chronic inflammation.

When the medical experts do look for the cause, they are usually all looking through a specific lens. If you are an anti-aging expert, you are looking for an increase in telomeres, the shoelace, like caps on the ends of DNA strands, which determines how long the cell is able to make copies of itself. Like the old saying, "If all you have is a hammer, everything looks like a nail." If by some method you increase telomere length, and you live longer, but you die of cancer, does it really matter how long your telomeres are? Or the fitness and weight loss plans that repeat the same old thought of *eat less and work out more*. This can be very difficult for someone who already has a slow metabolism, and in fact, research shows that this strategy increases stress on the body and further slows the metabolism. Not only will this approach slow metabolism, but it can also create hormonal imbalances and may lead to depression and/or anxiety.

Over the years, we have seen women suffering from hormonal imbalances for which some healthcare providers may prescribe birth control pills in order to help control their cycle or attempt to manage their hormones. If this fails, a hysterectomy can follow and then hormone replacement therapy for post-menopausal symptoms, neither of which may solve the original problem and has been found to possibly increase a person's risk for cancer.

Another example, low testosterone in men may lead to cardiovascular disease, diabetes, loss of muscle, loss of sex drive, and increased body fat. The standard remedy is to prescribe a medication to raise their testosterone, as opposed to looking for the cause of the low testosterone.

The body is not a collection of parts that work independently—it is a living system where all parts of the body are in communication with all the other parts of the body, both through chemical and electrical processes. Each part of the body affects the whole body. When things are out of balance, the body will do whatever is possible to bring it back into balance (homeostasis). An example of this is the pH of the blood; if the body becomes too acidic, it will release a hormone that causes calcium to be released from the bone into the bloodstream in order to bring it back to normal. The body has hundreds of processes like this that maintain homeostasis. Think of the body acting like a symphony orchestra. If the flute player is out of tune, everyone will hear it, including the conductor, and will want to make adjustments.

Your body operates perfectly, keeping you alive, in the present moment. Take, for instance, if you were to be attacked by a shark in the ocean. As you are bleeding, the blood flow would be diverted from all parts of the body that are not essential at that moment, because the brain needs the blood to stay alive. For example, the body will divert the blood from the kidneys to do this. If you survived for two weeks, you might die from kidney failure, but the body is not concerned with two weeks from now; it is only concerned with right now!

In this book, you will learn how to be the conductor of the symphony. The first part of the book identifies the systems of the body and how problems arise. The second part of the book discusses diets and dieting, and the third part advises you how to work toward correcting and enhancing your overall health.

In the following chapters, we will dive into the causes of stress and inflammation. We will discuss the physiology, symptoms, and after effects of stress on the body; and we will offer ways to decrease and mitigate these problems in order to help heal the body.

We hope you will also learn new concepts about health and wellness. The first concept we want to highlight is called the bioenergetic model of health. The main idea is that energy, function, and structure are interdependent at all levels of the body. What this means is that if the body or cell has enough energy and adequate metabolism, it can function properly, regenerate normally, and heal if damaged. However, if the body or the cell lacks energy, function will decrease to fit the available energy, and, more importantly, the cell will make abnormal copies of itself, causing aging and/or cancer.[1] It is important to note that if the cells are damaged, they will be unable to heal naturally and will be unable to restore normal function. Anything that slows energy or metabolism can cause "dis-ease" in the body.

Secondly, stress and inflammation lower energy and imbalance our hormones. Stress and inflammation are the cause of almost all disease processes that happen to the body. If we are to live healthy, happy lives, we must reduce or eliminate stress and inflammation.

Third, hormones dictate every process in the body. They control energy and metabolism. If we are to live productive, happy lives, we need to make sure our hormones are balanced.

## What We Have Learned From Covid-19

The spread and fatality rate of the coronavirus have put a spotlight on the state of health of not only America but also the rest of the world. Why is it that possibly 50% to 80% of the people infected are asymptomatic or exhibit just mild symptoms, but others are critically ill with high fatality rates?

What we know is that the elderly and people with comorbidities are affected much more than people that are young and "healthy." We are realizing that inflammation plays a significant role in determining whether we live or whether we die from this infection. As people age, it is known that inflammation rises. This "inflammaging" is the mechanism behind the development of cardiovascular disease, diabetes, obesity, autoimmune conditions, Hashimoto's thyroiditis, rheumatoid arthritis, lupus, psoriatic arthritis, and Alzheimer's disease. One of the major drivers of inflammation is chronic stress. We know stress is an immune system suppressor. Coupled with the effects of inflammation, it's the perfect storm that allows an opportunistic virus like COVID-19 to become a pandemic targeting those with pre-existing conditions and suboptimal states of general health. Other conditions that produce inflammation in the body are certain foods, chemicals, toxins, and pollution.[2]

This virus should be a wake-up call for our society to improve our health and shift the focus toward prevention and staying well rather than treatment of diseases already in progress. We can do a much better job at preventing pandemics by reducing stress and inflammation—rather than having to look for a new vaccine or novel drug therapy for each new virus that comes our way.

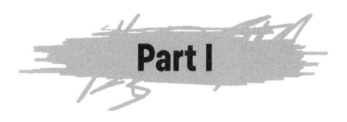

# Part I

## The Basics

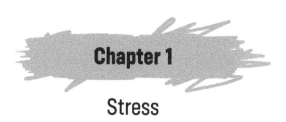

# Chapter 1

## Stress

What is stress? We all hear that stress is bad for you, but do you actually know what that means?

A concise definition of stress, and the one that we like to apply here, is "anything that raises the need for energy from baseline."

When we talk about stress, however, we are really talking about a stress response. This is also known as the "Fight, Flight, or Freeze Response." Let's use the classic example of getting chased by a lion: in this scenario, you are forced to either turn and fight, run away, or freeze in the hope that the lion races past you. When the stress response happens, it elicits a physiological cascade of events inside your body involving the autonomic nervous system. The autonomic nervous system controls all the functions of the body that are involuntary—blood pressure, breathing, heart rate, and blood flow.

There are two parts of the autonomic nervous system: (1) the *sympathetic* nervous system, known as the "fight or flight" system, which we just referenced, and (2) the *parasympathetic* nervous system, which is the "rest and digest" relaxation part of the nervous system. Under acute stress, the nervous system will divert the blood flow from your *gastrointestinal* (GI) tract to your skeletal muscles, so your body is able to fight or run or freeze. Heart rate and blood pressure will rise to supply more oxygen to the muscles to run and fight. Blood sugar will rise to supply the muscles with more energy. So, from our example of the lion chasing us, we are definitely needing more energy in order to escape the threat. In this situation, brain waves become faster and operate at a higher frequency in order to think about how to escape the threat—a stage referred to as *high Beta*. This higher frequency, in turn, leads to decreased problem-solving and lower creativity. Your thinking becomes narrowly focused as you are able to attend only to the threat at hand.

The stress response we just described is what we would call acute stress. By this we mean that the event happens, and we either get away from the lion or we become its dinner. The acute stress response is a natural response, and it's the way our bodies were designed: short bursts of stress that last just a few minutes, and then the body goes back to a normal state. If we are chased by the lion and get away, a short time later, the body's physiology has returned to normal, and we happily go about our day. Unfortunately, this is not the norm.

This acute stress response is a perfect response to keep us alive in the moment. The body, at that moment, is not worried about digesting food, making babies, long-term heart damage, growing hair, or repairing any damaged tissue. It is using all its resources in order to stay alive.

## Chronic Stress and Effects of Chronic Stress

For humans, the short-term stressor is not our main type of stress. As a species, we are more afflicted by chronic, long-term stress. What we mean by chronic stress is that it is not over within a few minutes, but actually goes on for hours, days, weeks, and even months. Many people that we have seen over the past twenty-five years are usually dealing with this type of ongoing stress.

Let's look at not only how this affects us but also what actually causes this chronic stress response. Remember that acute stress diverts blood flow from your gastrointestinal tract to your muscles. Chronic stress leads to impaired digestion due to a decrease in your stomach acid and a reduction in digestive enzymes. This, in turn, leads to stomach bloating, reflux, and heart burn. It is no coincidence that antacids and proton pump inhibitors (PPIs) like Nexium, "the purple pill," and Prilosec are some of the top-selling drugs in the world.[1] Chronic stress also decreases *peristalsis* (muscle contractions) of the intestines, which leads to chronic constipation.

Remember, blood pressure goes up with the stress response, and with chronic stress this leads to the development of *hypertension*, more commonly known as high blood pressure. The stress response also increases blood sugar which, of course, over time, if unregulated, can lead to Type 2 diabetes (NIDDM). Type 2 diabetes (non-insulin dependent diabetes mellitus) is an epidemic in the United States and worldwide. It has been reported that one-third of Americans and a growing number of other people throughout the world are either diabetic or prediabetic.[2]

Since stress (acute and especially chronic stress) uses more energy, the body has to pick and choose where it will maximize energy expenditure and where it will conserve energy. It's much like robbing Peter to pay Paul. The body starts turning off all non-essential body functions, for example, reproduction. Since the body knows that carrying a child to term is a drain on the woman's body, it will shut off the reproductive ability in order to conserve energy. So, not only does this chronic stress decrease a woman's ability to get pregnant, it also endangers the woman's ability to carry a pregnancy to term. And, guys, you don't get away in this department, either. It takes a lot of the body's energy to produce those little swimmers, so the body will reduce the sperm count and the sperm's viability. It often happens that a couple will try for years to get pregnant and maybe even try in vitro fertilization without success, but once they've given up trying to conceive, and the stress is eliminated, they finally become pregnant.

When talking about reproduction, we can't leave out reduced *libido* (sex drive). After working with thousands of patients, one of the biggest complaints we hear is not having a sex drive. It used to be a joke with men to say that their wife always had a headache, but there are just as many men as women with decreased libido. So, in essence, since most couples are dealing with chronic stress, they have become roommates instead of lovers.

Also, since the brain is one of the biggest energy consumers of the body, cognitive function is significantly reduced while suffering from chronic stress. This reduction actually causes loss of the *neurons* (nerve cells) to the part of the brain called the *hippocampus*, which plays an important role in learning and memory. This leads to memory problems, which play a role in the development of Alzheimer's disease.[3] Memory is not the only brain function that is affected. The frontal cortex also shows loss of neurons with chronic stress. The frontal cortex is the decision-making part of the brain—the impulse control center needed for long-term planning and gratification postponement.

It is no wonder people under stress have trouble at work coming up with solutions to problems, or that they often turn to alcohol, drugs, and/or gambling to find relief.

Now let's look at the effects of stress on the immune system. When you are running from the lion, your body is not thinking about using energy to make all the immune system chemicals. In fact, when a person has an organ transplant, doctors will give the person immunosuppressive drugs that mimic the stress response so the person does not reject the organ. When you are under stress, the body produces these hormones and chemicals and suppresses your own immune system.

Next, we have to look at the effects of chronic stress on weight gain. If you have ever taken, or ever known anyone who has taken, the anti-inflammatory/immunosuppressive drug *cortisone*, then you are aware of the weight gain and the classic moon face that goes along with taking it. Cortisone was created to mimic *cortisol*, one of the main stress hormones in the body. You just have to watch a little television to see all the ads attempting to sell you the latest and greatest "miracle supplements" that are supposed to block cortisol and eliminate "belly fat" (weight gain around the waist, hips, and/or stomach). The big pharma companies realize that cortisol is the main cause of weight gain, so many are researching and trying to bring to market cortisol blockers for weight loss.

One of the most detrimental effects of stress is the accelerated aging process. It has been shown that all the signs and symptoms of aging can be brought on by chronic stress. Studies show that chronic stress can damage cell DNA by shortening the telomeres. Telomeres are found on each end of the DNA strand and determine how many times the cell can copy itself.[4]

All these detrimental effects are precipitated by a release of hormones that produce these various responses to chronic stress. Most people have heard of the two main stress hormones, cortisol and adrenaline. Whenever you or anyone asks people what they know about cortisol, they answer, "It's the hormone that makes you get belly fat." And they are correct, but it actually does so much more than that. We will go into detail about how these two hormones work in the next chapter on hormones.

## Causes of Chronic Stress

We humans are rarely thinking in the present moment. We are ruminating over the past or anticipating the future or binge-watching our favorite show on Netflix or on our iPad. We are the only species that can elicit a stress response through our imagination. We can create that same fight or flight response just from our thoughts alone. So, when you are worrying about not enough money in the paycheck to pay the bills at the end of the month, or when you are worrying about meeting the deadline your boss has given you for that important project, you are producing the same chronic stress response and the same damaging stress hormones. How about when you're having relationship problems, wondering how to finance the children's college fund, worrying about how to care for an elderly parent, or when you're constantly trying to lose weight and it's not happening? The worry (stress) from any or all of these situations can be constant and ongoing—many times these stressors are with us twenty-four hours a day, day in and day out for years. This is how the mind creates true physical stressors from the issues or problems that we are often preoccupied with on a daily basis. One of the biggest contributors to chronic stress, believe it or not, is the food we eat and the "diet" we follow. This is a chapter unto itself because the food we eat—the diet we are following—is such a prevalent problem in our society, as evidenced by $72 billion spent on the diet industry every year.[5] Inflammation is a symptom of chronic stress from our diet, our environment, and other stressors.

Restricting calories is one of the major stressors on the body; it is like being in a famine. A famine is incredibly stressful and will cause our body to go into a stress mode. This can also happen if you do not take in the right macronutrients, proteins, carbs, and fats, or even the right micronutrients like vitamins and minerals. All of these things can shift our hormones out of balance. Interestingly, there's also the stress that healthy people bring on with certain types of exercise. We all know that exercise is good, but we have to know when it crosses over from healthy to destructive, and when it's actually causing harm instead of providing benefit. Many books will focus on the fact that the majority of people are not getting enough exercise; however, there can be too much of a good thing where exercise is concerned. We will go into great detail about this later in Part Three of this book.

What about all the environmental toxins and chemicals that we ingest from our food and absorb through our skin or breathe in through the air around us? The shampoos, body lotions, soaps, and chemicals that we come into contact with every day, and even the air we're breathing, can be a source of significant stress to the body. There are over 40,000 chemicals in the US market.[6] The EU has restricted or banned 1,300 chemicals in cosmetics, whereas the US has restricted only eleven chemicals.[7] This should be cause for concern.

And we can't forget about the importance of sleep and the stress response that occurs when a person is chronically sleep deprived or when their sleep cycle is suboptimal. Did you know that up to 70% of the people living in this country suffer from some form of sleep deprivation?[8] This can be a real game changer when corrected. If you're getting under seven to eight hours of sleep consistently, cortisol rises, and your body goes into chronic stress mode; let's just say that so many people in our population are not getting enough sleep.

The major causes of chronic stress go on and on. We will not cover all of them here. However, most of the major causes of chronic stress can be eliminated with the information we give you through our Eating Plan and our GI Plan.

Research shows us that chronic stress will eventually lead to the following diseases and conditions:

- diabetes
- obesity
- heart disease
- weakened immune system
- sexual dysfunction
- high blood pressure
- gastrointestinal issues
- respiratory infections
- insomnia
- fatigue
- depression
- anxiety
- autoimmune diseases[9]

This is just an overview of stress and the chronic stress response. In the next chapter, we will go over all the different hormones and their roles in the chronic stress response. The biggest takeaway here is that stress is the leading cause of weight gain, lower cognitive function, weakened immune system, anxiety, depression, and decreased sex drive. It is impossible to be healthy and productive if we do not have control over our stress response.

Parts Two and Three of this book are devoted to all the different ways that we can decrease, manage, and even eliminate the toxic effects of a chronic stress response.

---

## Takeaways from Chapter 1

1. Acute stress response is a natural response, but chronic stress leads to widespread damage throughout the body, the leading cause of weight gain, decreased cognitive function, a weakened immune system, disruption of hormone balance, and acceleration of the aging process.

2. Chronic stress is the number one factor behind many of the diseases/conditions we suffer with today.

3. One of the biggest contributors to chronic stress is the food we eat and the "diet" we follow, or the lack of adequate calories we consume.

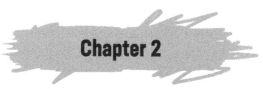

# Chapter 2

## Hormones Overview

When talking about health, wellness, and performance of the body, we rarely hear people mention hormones. It just doesn't make any sense not to mention hormones when you're talking about health, metabolism, mood, weight management, or optimal performance. Why do experts and researchers leave out hormones? Well, many researchers in the field of health and wellness have stated that hormones are just too complicated to discuss, so they tend to ignore them all together. Most experts, when they do talk about hormones, generally want to focus on one or another in particular.

However, this may be a great disservice when discussing our overall health. Hormones happen to be the most powerful chemicals in the body. There are dozens of hormones made in the body, each having a specific job to do. Tiny amounts of hormones measured in picograms and/or nanograms can have huge effects and, as such, are essential in any discussion around health, wellness, and optimal performance of the body.

In addition, it's important to understand that all hormones work together like a symphony orchestra, where each instrument is playing a vital and specific role, allowing for the overall outcome of a classic work of musical art (or optimal functioning of the body).

There is a scientific definition of a *hormone*, but an easier definition is, "a chemical produced in a gland secreted into the blood where it is transported to a target tissue."[1]

Hormones control metabolism, heart rate, blood pressure, reproduction, blood sugar, sex drive, mood, immune function, stress response, tissue growth, and the list goes on and on. Essentially, any and every bodily function you can think of is under the control of one or more hormones.

Consider driving your car: you don't need to know exactly how the engine and pistons work or how the transmission converts energy to the wheels to get where you want to go. In the same way, you don't need to know everything about hormones in order to function from day to day. However, a little knowledge will help you significantly improve your hormonal balance and your overall health.

In order to establish optimal health and wellness, it's important to have all of our hormones in balance. Although all hormones play a role in optimal health, for our purposes right now, we can focus on a few of the main stress hormones and still see significant improvements in our overall health. As we discuss these hormones, we will classify them as "good" and/or "bad" hormones; but, in reality, there are no "good" or "bad" ones—we need them all. Some hormones have a *catabolic* effect (breaking down). These can be considered the aging hormones, and they slow metabolism, which leads to storing fat. Some have an *anabolic* effect (building up). These can be considered the youth hormones and are primarily involved in increasing metabolism, which leads to loss of fat and building up of muscle. So, we want the aging hormones or fat-storing hormones to be as low as they can be within range, whereas we want the youth hormones or the fat-loss hormones to be as high as possible within range. The reason we want them still within range is that even the so-called "good" hormones, i.e., the youth hormones (anti-aging) or hormones focusing on building muscle/losing fat, can cause damage to the body if they are too high. The chart below shows some of the hormones we will focus on in this chapter and the chapters ahead:

| AGING Hormones | ANTI-AGING Hormones |
|---|---|
| Cortisol | Pregnenolone |
| Adrenaline (Epinephrine) | Progesterone |
| Estrogen | DHEA/Testosterone |
| Insulin | T4, T3 |

## Aging Hormones

- *Cortisol* is one of the main stress hormones.[2] It's produced by the adrenal gland as soon as there's any perceived stress—imagined or real. Any type of threat, situational, emotional, or even just the thought of something stressful, can elicit the stress response. Once this happens, cortisol is produced, enters the bloodstream, and sets off a whole cascade of events.

- *Adrenaline*—the other main stress hormone—is also produced by the adrenal gland and works in concert with cortisol.
- *Estrogen* is a fat-storing hormone, not only significant in women, but also significant in men. It causes cell proliferation, accelerates aging, and can be carcinogenic, causing uncontrolled cell growth, contributing to breast cancer in women and prostate cancer in men.
- *Insulin* allows glucose in the blood to get transported into the cell but becomes problematic when the cell becomes resistant to its effects.

## Anti-aging Hormones

- *Pregnenolone* is the precursor of two potent anti-aging hormones, DHEA and progesterone.
- *Progesterone* is actually the main female hormone. While the media and/or so-called "experts" will claim estrogen is the primary female hormone, progesterone is significantly more important in fertility, menstrual cycles, and menopause. It is anti-cancer and anti-estrogenic. It's not just for women, though, as men need and make progesterone, too.
- *DHEA* is considered the main anti-aging youth hormone. It works similar to testosterone. DHEA is also known as the "feel good" hormone, as it tends to help establish a sense of wellbeing and a more positive mood.
- *Testosterone* is a major anabolic (building) hormone—building muscle, fighting cancer, preventing heart disease, promoting good brain health, and managing blood sugar. Typically thought to be a predominantly male hormone, interestingly, women need adequate testosterone for optimal health, too.
- *Thyroid* hormones, T4 (*Thyroxine*) and T3 (*Triiodothyronine*), are the master metabolic hormones of the body, primarily involved in maintaining the body's energy level, important in maintaining a high metabolism.

## Takeaways from Chapter 2

1.  Hormones are responsible for all aspects of the body's function, not just reproduction.

2.  The anti-aging hormones are pregnenolone, progesterone, DHEA/testosterone, and thyroid hormones, T4 and T3.

3.  The aging hormones are cortisol, adrenaline, estrogen, and insulin.

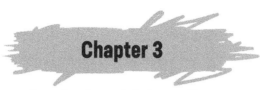

# Chapter 3

## Cortisol and Adrenaline

We have already mentioned the two aging/stress hormones, cortisol and adrenaline. So, let's go into some important facts about cortisol.

As previously pointed out, cortisol is a major stress hormone; however, since our bodies produce it, cortisol must have some significant benefits, too. The main purpose of cortisol during the stress response is to increase blood sugar as fuel in order to allow the muscles to function so you can carry out the appropriate fight or flight or freeze response.

If we didn't make cortisol, we would die.

Like all hormones, we need cortisol to be in range, because too much is bad, but not enough is equally as bad. The cortisol level needs to be within a certain range at certain times. For example, one of the most important functions of cortisol is creating glucose from our tissues when our blood sugar drops from lack of eating or not eating enough. We'll talk more about this in just a moment.

Cortisol also happens to be our main anti-inflammatory mediator in the body, so any time we have an injury or illness, cortisol levels will increase to bring down the inflammation; this is good in the short term but has detrimental effects if inflammation is an ongoing process. Also, timing is important when it comes to cortisol. There is a circadian rhythm to our cortisol levels. Cortisol is the hormone that wakes us up in the morning. It's produced in the adrenal glands, which are small, walnut-sized glands located on top of each kidney. When we look at a graph of daily cortisol levels, we see that it is high first thing in the morning, drops during the day, and is at its lowest levels in the evening.

This makes perfect sense, right? Cortisol is the ultimate stimulant—levels are highest in the mornings, when we want to be alert during the day, and lowest at night as we are going off to sleep. Some people who have been under stress for long periods of time or people who have a disrupted sleep cycle will have this graph reversed, meaning their cortisol levels will be low in the mornings and high in the evenings.

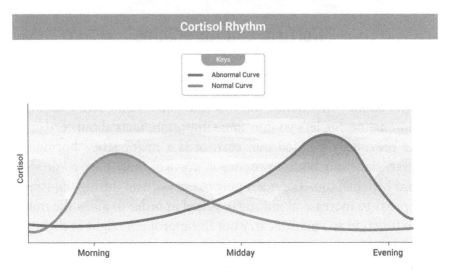

Figure 3.1. Cortisone is known as the wakeup hormone. Looking at normal daily cortisone levels, it is high first thing in the morning to wake us up, continually drops during the day, and then is at the lowest levels in the evening when we are ready to go to sleep.

These are the people who cannot get to sleep at night and cannot get up in the morning. When they are trying to sleep, they feel "wound up" and run down at the same time. They are the people who are living on caffeine to get through the day. Sound familiar? A vast majority of Americans can't start their day without coffee. This is why caffeine is the number-one selling, legalized drug in the world.

Remember how we said that cortisol is the ultimate stimulant? Well, it can also wake you in the night, if your blood sugar levels fall. If this happens, in the middle of the night, the body will release cortisol to raise the blood sugar levels. And since cortisol is the wakeup hormone, your body thinks it's time to get up—even though it is only two o'clock a.m.! The next time you're lying in bed awake in the middle of night staring at the ceiling, you'll understand the reason why.

There are two major medical conditions involving cortisol levels, one in which the cortisol levels are too high and one in which the cortisol levels are too low. With cortisol levels that are too low, the adrenal glands are not producing enough cortisol. This is called *Addison's disease*—a rather rare disease (it is what President John F. Kennedy suffered with for years). This condition required him to take cortisol every day to function. Cortisone is also known as *prednisone*. Some of the symptoms of Addison's disease, (if left untreated) are the following:

- irritability
- depression
- anxiety
- mood swings
- body hair loss
- extreme fatigue
- weight loss
- decreased appetite
- darkening skin (*hyperpigmentation*)
- low blood pressure
- salt craving
- nausea
- diarrhea
- abdominal pain
- muscle or joint pains
- sexual dysfunction
- low blood sugar (*hypoglycemia*)

The second disease, which is far more common, is when cortisol levels are too high. This is called *Cushing's syndrome*, sometimes referred to as *hypercortisolism*. Cushing's syndrome can happen after taking a prolonged course of oral corticosteroids, like prednisone, or it can happen when your body produces too much cortisol on its own. When your body produces too much cortisol on its own, the cause is usually a pituitary tumor, but this condition can be caused by the adrenal gland itself. Many times, healthcare providers aren't usually addressing excess cortisol levels until they get to a pathological level, despite the damage that occurs with even moderately increased cortisol levels over time. Some of the symptoms of Cushing's syndrome are the following:

- weight gain—particularly around the midsection and upper back

- the face becomes full (often referred to as "moon face")
- a hump between the shoulders (often referred to as a "buffalo hump")
- purple stretch marks on abdomen, thighs, breasts, and/or arms
- thinning skin that bruises easily
- thicker or more visible body and facial hair (*hirsutism*)
- irregular menstrual periods
- low libido
- erectile dysfunction (ED)
- decreased fertility
- fatigue
- muscle weakness
- depression
- anxiety
- cognitive difficulties, like "brain fog"
- increased pigmentation of the skin—especially the neck, groin, and armpits

These can be common symptoms of Cushing's syndrome, but if you are under significant stress and have high cortisol levels for extended periods of time, you can have the exact same symptoms.

Whenever we are under stress, whether we are being chased by the lion or worrying about too many bills; if the stress is ongoing, it will start the cascade of stress hormones. As noted above, the negative effects can be catastrophic.

Going back to our classic example of getting chased by a lion, we talked about the physical responses of the body to acute and chronic stress. These stress responses are mainly due to increased cortisol levels, which actually come from a coordinated response from the central nervous system. What happens when that lion chases you or when you are constantly thinking about that deadline at work? This information is sent to a part of the brain called the *amygdala*. It oversees emotional processes such as fear and anxiety. When the amygdala interprets this information as a threat, it then sends a distress signal to another part of the brain called the *hypothalamus*.

The hypothalamus is like the command center for the brain. It communicates with the rest of the body through a complex circuitry of nerves/neurons, the *autonomic nervous system*. The hypothalamus utilizes another gland, the pituitary, as its main messaging center. The *pituitary* is a pea-sized gland referred to as the "master gland," and it is responsible for secreting many of the hormones that we will talk about in this book. Cortisol is not the only stress hormone. There's another key player in the stress response, adrenhaline.

Initially, the response from the hypothalamus is to send a signal through the autonomic nerves, bypassing the pituitary all the way to the adrenal glands to release *epinephrine*, more commonly known as adrenaline. This response can happen quickly, even before you realize that there is any danger. This allows you to react without even thinking. The adrenal glands start pumping adrenaline into the bloodstream, which causes the heart to beat faster to send more blood to the heart and other vital organs. This will in turn increase the breathing rate to create more oxygen in the blood. More oxygen in the bloodstream allows for the brain to be more alert for the threat at hand. Increased adrenaline allows for the muscles to work harder to either run away from the threat or stay and fight. Adrenaline also heightens hearing, sight, and other senses.

While this initial surge of adrenaline is subsiding, the amygdala activates another important part of this system through the pituitary gland. The hypothalamus, the pituitary, and the adrenal glands form a complex and highly sophisticated stress response center known as the *hypothalamus–pituitary–adrenal axis* (HPA). The HPA axis runs like any big corporation. The hypothalamus acts like the CEO in the company—he/she doesn't usually communicate directly with the employees but achieves the company's operational plan by working through intermediate managers to communicate the directives and work objectives to the employees. You can think of the pituitary and adrenal glands as the intermediate managers and the individual hormones as the employees. The HPA axis uses hormones to keep the stress response going. The hypothalamus, as the command center, releases *corticotropin-releasing hormone*, CRH for short. CRH signals the pituitary gland to release another key player, *adrenocorticotropic hormone*, or ACTH for short. ACTH signals the adrenal gland to produce both cortisol and adrenaline, and the cycle begins again.

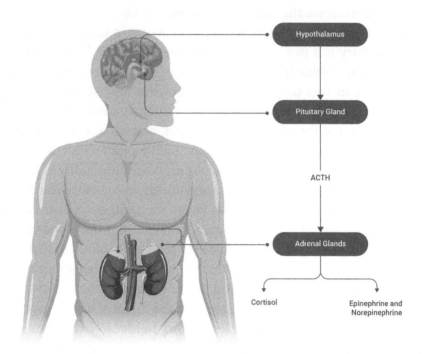

Figure 3.2. Our body's stress response center, the HPA axis, is made up of the hypothalamus, the pituitary, and the adrenal glands. The HPA axis uses hormones to keep our stress response going.

Many people are running around with high levels of adrenaline in a constant state of stress. This is what activates and maintains an ongoing response of the HPA axis. The HPA axis was never intended for chronic activation. Chronic activation means chronic stress, and this causes significant issues throughout the body, as we have been discussing. Once the stressful event is over, then the other part of the central nervous system—the *parasympathetic system*—will take over and calm the stress response down. The problem is with chronic stressors, most of us will never reach this stage where the stressful response is over.

Now, we will transition from neuroscience to some basic biochemistry to understand the body's stress response at the lowest level. The process of raising blood sugar levels is done through the biochemical reaction called *gluconeogenesis*. This big intimidating word is easy to understand once we break it down. The first part of the word comes from the word "glucose" because this is the sugar molecule that is the preferred energy source of the body. The next part is "neo," which means "new," and the last part is "genesis," which means "production." Altogether, this word describes the process of producing new glucose. Your body will create glucose (sugar) by breaking down protein.

Where does the body get the protein? It actually comes from breaking down tissues—mainly in muscle, organs, and glands. We think you will agree that this doesn't sound good, right? We all want more muscle; we don't want less, and we definitely don't want the muscle we have to be broken down in order to serve as the primary source of energy for the body!

When cortisol breaks down organs and/or glands, one of the most affected glands is the thymus gland. This gland is located just under your breastbone (sternum). This gland is important because it is one of the major components of the immune system. One of the immune system's key defenses is the T cell. These T cells originate as immature, immune precursor cells from the bone marrow and then travel through the bloodstream to the thymus gland, where they mature into active T cells. T cells have a variety of functions within the immune system, one of which is fighting cancer and other foreign invaders such as bacteria, viruses, and parasites. It was thought at one time that the thymus gland shrinks as we age because autopsies performed on elderly people often showed small to nonexistent thymus glands. However, more current research reveals that the gland had decreased in size due to illness or stress, resulting in a crippled and significantly impaired immune system. When everyone talks about stress as a killer, this is actually what they're talking about. The good news is that, with the right protocols, the thymus gland can be regenerated.[1]

We just talked about where cortisol breaks down protein, but it also breaks down fat. That's got to be good news, right? Sorry—the fat that it breaks down is mainly from the periphery like the arms and the legs, but cortisol actually stores visceral fat around the waist area and around other organs, which is not good. A classic body type as a result of this is a big belly and thinner arms and legs. Visceral fat will create a lot of inflammation, and this, in turn, causes more cortisol production in a never-ending loop. We will tell you how to lose the visceral fat in the second half of the book.

Both cortisol and adrenaline can cause *lipolysis*, which is the process of breaking down fat. "Lipo" means "fat" and "lysis" means "breaking down." This means that both cortisol and adrenaline break down the peripheral fat that is stored in the body and release *free fatty acids* into the bloodstream for energy (FFAs for short). Losing body fat is a good thing if we lose it slowly and if we do not overwhelm the body with a lot of free fatty acids in the bloodstream all at one time. Remember the term free fatty acids, as this will be important later when we talk about dietary sources of chronic inflammation. More about all of this when we talk about the role of inflammation in diet and weight loss.

The body will release cortisol and adrenaline to form glucose and to release fat so the body can have a significant energy source. Too many free fatty acids in the bloodstream prevent glucose from being utilized by the cells and, as a result, will cause glucose to increase in the bloodstream. We will cover all of this and more in the chapter on insulin. These aging/stress hormones—cortisol and adrenaline—also affect many other hormones. For example, as cortisol levels rise, two other stress/aging hormones—insulin and estrogen—increase, and the anabolic/anti-aging hormones—pregnenolone, progesterone, testosterone, T4, and T3—all decrease. It is much like the seesaw that you played on as a child: When one side goes up, the other side goes down. At this point, you can realize how important it is to keep the stress response and the stress hormones, i.e., cortisol and adrenaline, at low levels.

When we talk about stress, we must also talk about our diet. As we mentioned earlier, dieting is a significant stressor. Really, one of the most stressful events for the body is dieting and starvation, which, believe it or not, is a common problem among Americans today. Most people think of weight loss as requiring limited calories and increased exercise. You may hear people telling you, possibly even your healthcare provider, that to lose the weight, you need to "eat less and workout more".

However, when a person eats fewer calories than they need, they are actually in starvation mode, which is a huge stress to the body. When you do not have enough glucose or stored glucose (glycogen) available, the body interprets this as a time of famine. The response then is to slow the metabolism to preserve calories. And to do this, the body uses muscle as its preferred energy source and stored fat as a last resort.

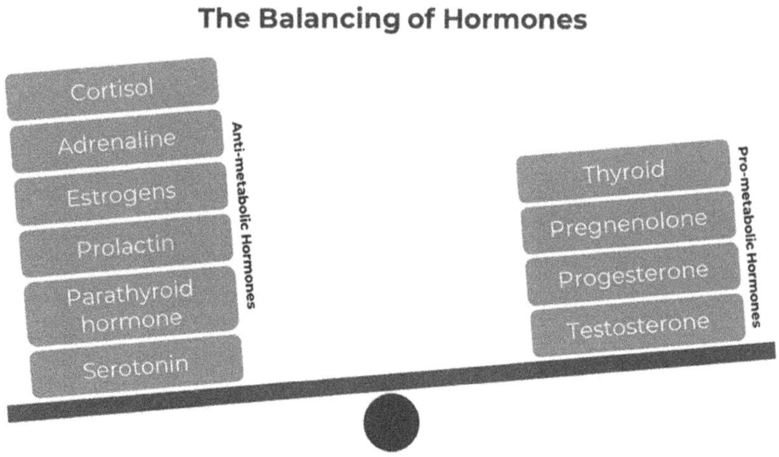

## The Balancing of Hormones

Figure 3.3. The stress hormones cortisol and adrenaline affect other hormones. As their levels rise, aging hormones increase, while anti-aging hormones decrease, tipping the scales of your hormonal balance.

Weight loss is much more than the common knowledge of "calories in versus calories out" theory of weight loss. Weight loss is actually more about hormones and energy than about dieting and exercise. If you think about it, you intuitively know it's about hormones because when you were fifteen years old, you could eat a whole box of Fruit Loops and not gain an ounce, but now, you might count out twelve Cheerios and put on a pound. This is one of the most important lifestyle aspects that we can control and affect. We will do a deep dive into diet in the second part of this book.

## Takeaways from Chapter 3

1. Cortisol and adrenaline are the main stress hormones and cause an increase in aging hormones, while decreasing anti-aging hormones.

2. Cortisol is our main anti-inflammatory mediator—levels rise to fight inflammation.

3. Chronic activation of the hypothalamus-pituitary-adrenal axis means chronic stress response and the widespread damages that go with it.

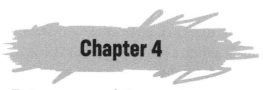

# Chapter 4

## Estrogen and Progesterone

### Estrogen Is Not Just a Problem for Women

Even though it is considered the female hormone, men, you have it too. In fact, some middle-aged men have as much estrogen as middle-aged women. Even the young men of today have high levels of estrogen due to excess hormone disrupters in food and chemicals, increased body fat, and poor diets.[1] These are not the only reasons, though. We'll be talking about this subject throughout this chapter. Often, older men with high levels of estrogen have a distinctive odor about them. So, this chapter on estrogen is for you, men, too.

Estrogen may be the most misunderstood hormone by conventional allopathic medicine. The current climate of biomedical hormone replacement therapy is confusing to people for many reasons. It's difficult to get a clear consensus among today's healthcare providers. This is demonstrated by increases in all female cancers,[2] strokes, blood clots, and weight gain, most notably since the beginning of the approval of Premarin,* an estrogen derivative obtained from pregnant mares used for women in menopause.[3]

The hormone estrogen has been touted as "the female hormone" for nearly a hundred years. At first, it was used for "female problems," then it was used for improving fertility, then it was used as a form of birth control, and more recently as a biomedical hormone replacement therapy. But since the 1950s, researchers have been aware of its toxic effects.

Currently, estrogen is given to women who are menopausal to prevent osteoporosis and to help with hot flashes. It is also given to women who are cycling and having menstrual "problems." The medical community has repeatedly dismissed the increased risk of developing breast and ovarian cancers that have been shown to be associated with the use of estrogen replacement therapy. Only after a woman has developed cancer does she then receive drugs to block estrogen. With our current medical model, estrogen has been condoned for medical use, then after causing disease, it is viewed as a problem. Many healthcare providers see the benefits as outweighing the risks in developing subsequent breast and ovarian cancers; they seem to promote the advantages of estrogen over its more problematic and/or lethal effects.[4] It would be like giving you poison first and then giving you the antidote. The continuing use of estrogen for osteoporosis is puzzling, even after a large research study completed in 2005 called The Women's Health Initiative (WHI) showed that estrogen was neither the cause nor the cure for bone loss. The Women's Health Initiative happens to be the largest research study ever funded by the NIH. Budgeted at $625 million over fourteen years, the study was designed to test strategies to prevent cardiovascular disease, breast cancer, and osteoporotic fractures—leading causes of death, disability, and decreased quality of life for older women. [5] Why, then, is estrogen prescribed by almost every gynecologist/primary healthcare provider? Why else? Like many things, there has been a lot of favourable advertising by the pharmaceutical companies for which this is a very big money maker.

## Okay, Men: You Can Skip the Following Section

In order to better understand the role of estrogen in health and inflammation, we need to talk more about the details of a woman's menstrual cycle. Estrogen is low until about day thirteen or fourteen of the cycle, and then suddenly, there is a huge spike in estrogen. This is the signal to release the egg from the ovary. Then estrogen will decrease as progesterone rises, which allows for the egg to implant in the uterus and for the fetus to become viable. Progesterone allows the pregnancy to come to term. If progesterone does not rise and/or estrogen levels remain high, then the mother will most likely spontaneously abort the fetus. If the mother does not become pregnant, then progesterone levels fall, the uterine lining sloughs off, and the whole cycle starts over. This is the reason why fertility doctors prescribe progesterone to women who have conceived and who have a prior history of miscarriages: to ensure that the pregnancy goes to term.

Let's look at the effects that estrogen has on the body. We spoke about how it's the signal to release the egg for fertilization, but it does much more for the rest of the body. Most women are aware of the bloating that comes along with ovulation and can occur at other times when their cycle is "off." Excess estrogen in combination with inflammatory mediators increases vascular leakiness and causes the cells to take up calcium and water. This leads to edema and swelling.

Many women through the years have experiencedt fertility problems. They have had high estrogen levels and low progesterone levels when tested and were told that they were unable to conceive or would have a miscarriage if they tried to get pregnant. Once the hormones become balanced, meaning low estrogen and high progesterone, women would become fertile and then conceive easily without any need for in vitro fertilization or any other damaging fertility drugs. A woman's fertility is a direct result of a healthy body and balanced hormones.

We think it is much better to address imbalances in estrogen/progesterone than to try to force the woman's body to conceive when it is not healthy. This is the beauty of the innate wisdom of the body.

In reality, many women are estrogen dominant: either the body is producing too much estrogen relative to progesterone, or the body is not producing enough progesterone relative to estrogen. So, what are some of the symptoms of a woman who is estrogen dominant? In our practices, we hear the following symptoms from most women. Most of the time they have been treated by their primary healthcare provider or gynecologist without resolving any of these issues.

Excess estrogen symptoms include the following:
- weight gain
- edema/swelling
- infertility
- varicose veins
- mood swings
- depression/anxiety
- breast tenderness
- irregular cycles
- heavy cycles/missed cycles
- insomnia
- night sweats
- fatigue
- benign cysts/fibrocystic breast disease

- breast cancer
- lower metabolic rate
- darkened pigmentation of skin, usually up around the neck area
- decrease elasticity of skin
- lower body temperature
- bloating
- PMS
- headaches/migraines
- blood clots/thromboembolism

The most prevalent symptoms of estrogen dominance are heavy and/or irregular periods. Many will have shortened cycles or even multiple cycles within a month. Most will say the flow is heavy, with clots and preceded by cramps. Estrogen causes the uterine lining to become thickened, and so, when it sloughs off, this will produce heavy bleeding, clots, and cramps. The conventional medical model to treat these symptoms is to give birth control pills.[6] This is just like pouring gas on the fire because, now, you've just given more estrogen to a woman already making too much. This may make the cycle more predictable but will not solve any of the other symptoms such as bloating, weight gain, PMS, low libido, swelling ankles, or the other symptoms she is dealing with.

If you're not sure whether or not this is true, just look at the warnings on the insert of one estradiol birth control pill: Atrial fibrillation, cerebrovascular disease, coronary artery disease, coronary thrombosis, edema, endocarditis, hypercholesterolemia, hypertension, myocardial infarction, renal disease, stroke, thromboembolic disease, thromboembolism, thrombophlebitis, valvular heart disease.

In the rare case that your healthcare provider performs a laboratory test to measure hormones, the great majority of the time, they will test for only estrogen. When testing for estrogen, there are three types of estrogen metabolites: estradiol, estrone, and estriol. One of the biggest problems is that most of the estrogen is stored in the body's tissues and not in the blood. In fact, some studies show up to one hundred times difference between blood and body tissue estrogen levels.[7] This means the only way to get an accurate measurement would be to do a tissue biopsy, but this is invasive and, therefore, not practical.[8] The second problem with testing just estrogen is that the progesterone-to-estrogen ratio is far more important than each hormone level individually. This means that you could have estrogen at the high end of the normal range and progesterone at the low end of the normal range—but, the ratio would show estrogen dominance, even though both are within normal range. Also, depending on the day of the month, these levels can change dramatically and will fluctuate. Reviewing symptoms is much easier and can be more accurate in addressing these problems than looking at lab values.[9]

If the birth control pill is not the answer, then how do we make estrogen dominance better, and how do we level out these hormone imbalances? One of the main culprits behind estrogen dominance is increased cortisol and adrenaline, which, as mentioned earlier, are mass-produced during the chronic stress response. Imbalances in the other hormones we talked about in Chapter 2 can also create estrogen excess. We will be working through lifestyle changes, dietary supplements, and other natural ways to correct and restore a more beneficial estrogen/progesterone balance. So, this discussion is important for cycling females and those that are having issues with excess estrogen. However, some of you are menopausal, and your healthcare provider may have put you on estrogen for hot flashes, low libido, insomnia, thinning vaginal wall, and incontinence. This may be helping the hot flashes for a short time, but rarely do we see it improving any of the other menopausal symptoms.

Consider this explanation: "But the doctor told me since my ovaries are not working, that I do not produce estrogen anymore" or "this is early onset menopause from a hysterectomy, I don't make estrogen anymore". This is not entirely true. For one thing, the predominant focus on estrogen is because estrogen is a billion-dollar business. When a woman enters menopause, the ovaries cease production of both estrogen and progesterone. However, most of the hormone decrease is actually progesterone, not estrogen.

The adrenal glands will produce a small amount of progesterone. But note that, in the context of talking about the chronic stress response, production of progesterone through the adrenal gland will be greatly diminished. Therefore, the hormonal symptoms of menopause are not necessarily caused by a huge drop in estrogen, but more accurately by a dramatic loss of progesterone. We will talk about the importance and benefits of maintaining a high level of progesterone in a separate section.

One of the most detrimental effects of estrogen is how it accelerates the aging process. Increased estrogen levels inhibit the production of carbon dioxide, which is essential to adequate oxygenation of the body's tissues. Oxygen deprivation in the tissues leads to a process called *lipid peroxidation*. Lipid peroxidation is a toxic process whereby fats are broken down and free radicals are produced. These free radicals do a lot of damage to cells and tissues. Excess estrogen in the tissues also increases fibrotic changes in connective tissue, which makes the skin less elastic and accelerates pigmentation of the skin and organs.[11] Have you noticed the brown age spots people get as they get older? Excess estrogen will also lower body temperature, cause crepiness in the skin, increase the formation of blood clots, and cause the thymus gland to decrease in size, which, in turn, will lower immune system function and increase the probability for autoimmune disorders.

## Okay, Men: This Is Also for You

A recent study shows that, at least in women, excess estrogen is closely associated with the general loss of fat-free tissue with aging—meaning they lose muscle and collagen instead of fat.[12]

There are certain enzymes that produce estrogen in the body's tissues. One is known as *aromatase* (also called *estrogen synthase*). Aromatase converts some of the body's building hormones into estrogen. It is an enzyme that is found in all parts of the body, male and female. The skin and fat are major sources of aromatase, and the levels increase with age and body fat.[13] The older we get, and the more fat we accumulate, the more estrogen we will produce. This excess estrogen causes more fat, which produces more aromatase, and the whole process becomes a never-ending cycle.

A class of drugs known as *aromatase inhibitors*, which block the production of estrogen in women and men, have now become a common pharmaceutical target in the treatment of breast cancer.[14] Aromatase inhibitors are also used with men who are on testosterone replacement therapy in order to block the testosterone they are receiving from being converted into estrogen.

Men produce estrogen also, just not as much as women. Just like women, as men age, their body fat increases, causing an increase in aromatase activity, and this creates excess estrogen. The aromatase will take a man's testosterone and DHEA and convert it into estrogen. This is why some middle-aged men may actually have as much estrogen as middle-aged women. The telltale signs of excess estrogen in men are weight gain, loss of muscle mass, cardiovascular conditions, "man boobs," "love handles," erectile dysfunction, and loss of libido. Another condition of excess estrogen in men is a condition known as *benign prostatic hypertrophy* (BPH), which refers to an enlarged prostate, present in about 90% of men by the age of eighty years old.[15]

This condition will lead to increased urination, especially at night. Eventually, excess estrogen can lead to prostate cancer. Symptoms that we described above referring to excess estrogen, at one time, used to be signs associated with old age, but now we see these in young men and even teenagers. Back then, excess estrogen was a sign of aging poorly.

There are a few predominant reasons for this trend—namely, the effects of chronic stress in today's busy lifestyle, the effects of chemicals in the food we eat (like pesticides and preservatives), chemicals present in water bottles that we are drinking out of, chemicals present in the food storage containers and cookware that we are eating from, and even chemicals that we put on our skin. These chemicals act like estrogen and are significant hormone disrupters. There's a particular class of hormone disrupter referred to as *phytoestrogens*, and they are everywhere, in the food we eat and products that we apply to our skin.[16]

Back to our discussion on the toxic effects of chronic stress: stress causes increased estrogen, and increased estrogen causes stress. An example of this would be male runners who often double their estrogen levels after running a marathon. It has been noted that both men and women who have been hospitalized with a serious illness often show increased estrogen levels.

Let's summarize estrogen:
- estrogen is a fat-storing hormone
- estrogen increases the risk of cancer[17]
- estrogen suppresses the immune system

- estrogen accelerates the aging process[18]
- excess estrogen causes edema/swelling, mood changes, fatigue, insomnia, night sweats, lowered libido, and the list goes on and on[19]

The main takeaway here for both men and women is that we want to keep estrogen levels low. You can do this naturally through some basic lifestyle choices with your diet, with supplements, with sleep, and with your breathing techniques. A popular movement right now, bio-hacking, is defined as the practice of changing our physiology and chemistry through science and self-experimentation to enhance the body.[20]

---

### Takeaways from Chapter 4

1. Estrogen dominance is a significant cause of many problems women experience today. Men can have elevated estrogen levels, too, not just women.

2. Although we think of menopause as a significant drop in estrogen levels, it is more accurately brought on by a dramatic drop in progesterone.

3. Stress causes increased estrogen, and increased estrogen causes stress; therefore, for both men and women, the important goal is keeping estrogen levels low.

---

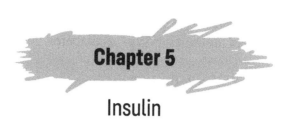

# Chapter 5

## Insulin

In the last chapter, we were talking about estrogen. So, to continue with the aging and stress hormones, we will now discuss the hormone *insulin* and attempt to dispel some prevalent and common misunderstandings about this particular hormone. Almost everyone has heard about the hormone insulin. It's mentioned in all the commercials about diabetes—the ones about medications that are being shown on network television every few minutes, or so it seems. This is a hormone around which there seems to be a lot of confusion. Most people might understand that too much insulin is not good, but the role of insulin is to decrease the amount of blood sugar in the bloodstream; but, if you have high levels of insulin and high blood sugar, this is not good, either. Isn't this a contradiction? How do we know if insulin is really the problem?

Insulin is one of the main hormones related to blood sugar; it helps your cells take up glucose to be used for fuel. As we mentioned earlier when we were talking about cortisol and adrenaline, at rest, your muscles will mainly use fat as a local source of energy, but with a chronic and ongoing stress response or with high-intensity exercise, your muscles will switch to glucose as their preferred energy source.

The hormone insulin is produced and released by cells called beta (β) cells, located in the pancreas. One of its primary purposes is to help the body regulate blood sugar. If your pancreas is unable to make insulin, or if the levels of insulin the pancreas is producing are suboptimal, this can create a condition referred to as Type 1 diabetes. It used to be called (and some people still use the term) "juvenile diabetes," referring to its predominance in children.

However, Type I diabetes can also occur in adults. In both cases, it is usually an auto-immune condition in which the body actually attacks and destroys its own beta (β) cells in the pancreas. One particular patient had developed Type 1 diabetes after contracting a virus in one eye. The virus migrated to the pancreas and caused the destruction of beta (β) cells through the overactivation of the immune system. A Type 1 diabetic must take insulin medication for the rest of their life, or they will die. Though this is a profoundly serious disease, we will focus on the more prevalent disease in our society, and that is the one caused mainly by a sedentary lifestyle, chronic stress, and poor diet. This type of diabetes is referred to as Type 2 diabetes. Since this is mainly a lifestyle disease, this means there are many things we can do to change it, and even better, to prevent it and reverse it.[1] Type 2 diabetes, also known *as insulin resistance*, is an epidemic in westernized society. You may have heard the term "adult-onset diabetes," named because it predominantly affects adults.

With our changing diets and our more sedentary and chronically stressful lifestyles, diabetes is becoming more prevalent in younger people, including children. According to the Centers for Disease Control *National Diabetes Statistics Report 2020*, the statistics for diabetes (Type 1 and Type 2) suggest that around thirty-four million people in the US have diabetes; some statistics project that around seven million people have diabetes but have not yet been diagnosed, with the majority of these being Type 2 diabetics. The number of prediabetics is estimated at eighty-eight million people, with thirty to fifty% of these going on to develop full-blown Type 2 diabetes. This means that, using these statistics, approximately one-third of the US population has some sort of problem related to blood sugar regulation. In this chapter, the terms "glucose" and "sugar" are interchangeable. However, they are not necessarily synonymous; when we get into the discussion of diet, we'll be using the terms "carbohydrates" and "sugar" as a more inclusive category.

Let's look at some of the effects of Type 2 diabetes, resulting from having chronic high blood sugar levels, which contributes to or directly causes the following:

- obesity
- damaged blood vessels
- heart disease/heart attack
- stroke

- kidney damage/failure
- eye damage/loss of vision
- nerve problems
- sexual dysfunction/erectile dysfunction
- Alzheimer's disease/dementia—now thought of as Type 3 diabetes
- slow healing wounds that can lead to amputations

To better understand the concept of insulin resistance, we can use the analogy of a lock and a key. If, for example, you want to get in the front door of your house while the door is locked, you'll need your key to unlock the door, and then you can walk right in. But what happens if your key doesn't fit the lock or if the lock is broken? You won't get inside. This is pretty much how insulin resistance works. Insulin resistance occurs when the insulin receptor on any cell (i.e., the lock) loses its sensitivity to insulin (i.e., the key), and when the key doesn't fit the lock, or the lock does not recognize the key, the glucose cannot enter the cell to serve as a source of energy. Our main goal concerning insulin, then, is to restore the sensitivity of the insulin receptor (i.e., fix the lock), so that it takes little effort to allow the glucose into the cell.

This is an extremely important topic, as many people today are being treated for diabetes, and even prediabetes, without fully understanding what's really happening. There's often confusion around the idea of insulin resistance versus insulin sensitivity. We want you to remember that the more sensitive the cells in the body are to insulin, the easier it is to remove the glucose from the bloodstream and get it into the cell for processing.

Since the Type 2 diabetic cell has become less sensitive to insulin, the body must work harder to get the glucose into the cell. The more resistant the cells, the more insulin is required for this to happen. The longer this goes on, the more and more insulin it takes to get the glucose into the cell. Insulin resistance results in increasingly higher levels of blood sugar in the bloodstream over time.

Now here is where we may go against all conventional wisdom by the so-called experts, medical dogma, and mainstream media.

# Hormone Receptor

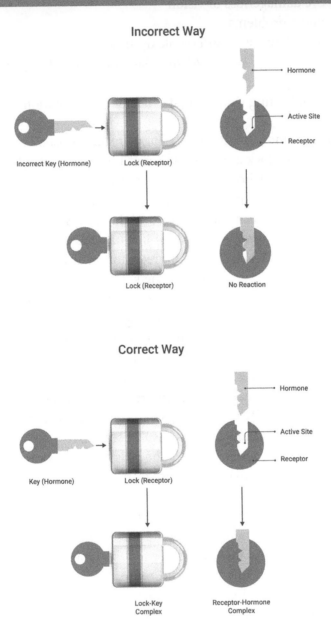

Figure 5.1. Insulin resistance occurs when the insulin receptor on any cell (i.e., the lock) loses its sensitivity to insulin (i.e., the key), and when the key doesn't fit the lock or the lock does not recognize the key, the glucose cannot enter the cell to serve as a source of energy.

What does everyone say is the cause of insulin resistance? They say it's sugar, right? Or the intake of carbs, which eventually all break down to sugar. But this is actually the wrong answer. Insulin resistance and high blood sugar are symptoms of a bigger problem, but not the cause. If you have a clogged kitchen sink and water isn't going down the drain, you don't say that the water is the problem and shut the water off to the house. That does nothing to correct the problem. The mainstay of managing diabetes today is limiting sugar intake and attempting to regulate blood sugar levels. And because sugar is actually not the problem, it is illogical to try to heal the body by managing these symptoms. So, hang in here while we explain. This is one of the most important concepts for your overall health and optimal wellness. It's not as simple as just eating less sugar or eating fewer carbs.

Unfortunately, you can often hear from healthcare professionals or even from the medical media that the cell is "too full of sugar" (i.e., glucose). This is their explanation for how the cell becomes resistant to insulin. However, this is not how the biochemistry of the body works. Although we will not give a dissertation on biochemistry here, just know that sugar (i.e., glucose) is transported into the cell to create energy in a complicated three-step process: Step 1—glycolysis, Step 2—Krebs cycle, and Step 3—the electron transport chain.

The end-product of this three-step process is actually energy produced in the form of a molecule known as *adenosine triphosphate* (ATP). In fact, we know that people who are diabetic through insulin resistance are actually suffering from too little energy production in the cell because the glucose concentrations in the cell are too low. This is because with insulin resistance, as we mentioned above, it becomes difficult to get the glucose from the bloodstream into the cell. Any cellular function that needs glucose or energy to function will be impaired, even though the blood glucose/sugar levels may remain high.

Let's summarize the insulin response. When we eat carbohydrates, they break down into glucose, and the glucose circulates through the bloodstream. The body senses a rise in the blood sugar level and releases insulin from the beta (β) cells of the pancreas. The insulin then reacts by way of a specific receptor on the cell that allows the glucose into the cell. The glucose in the cell is then to be converted into energy in the form of ATP.

When only small amounts of insulin are needed to allow glucose into the cell for this energy-producing process, we call this insulin sensitivity. This is a good thing. However, if the cell receptor is unresponsive to insulin and glucose is unable to enter the cell, then blood sugar levels will rise. We call it insulin resistance now, as it represents cells all throughout the body that have become resistant to the effects of insulin. When the cells' receptors become unresponsive to the insulin, the body will manufacture more in an attempt to try to overwhelm the receptor and force the glucose into the cell. The pancreas has to release more and more insulin now to allow the receptor to take up the glucose.

At this stage, a person is often started on a common medication, usually metformin, to aid in the cells' uptake of glucose. This may help to manage the rising blood sugar levels, but it does not "cure" or really even address the underlying problem that the cells' receptors are resistant to insulin.[2] Metformin is like all other diabetic medications on the market today: it acts as a band-aid but does not "fix" the underlying problem. Eventually, many people will continue to have high blood sugar levels, and the pancreas will no longer be able to keep up with the demand. When this happens, the person is then given insulin. An important distinction: Type 1 diabetics cannot make insulin. Type 2 diabetics can still make insulin. The medical community approaches high blood sugar as if, "we just cut out carbs, or limit sugar intake, then we have fixed the problem." But will this actually lower the blood sugar levels? And does that really matter? Sometimes, it does. However, this "fix" does little, if anything, to correct the underlying problem—namely, the receptors' insensitivity to the insulin. This only means that whenever the person eats carbs again, they return to having high blood sugar circulating throughout the bloodstream, and high blood sugar levels in the bloodstream lead to all the short/long-term effects of diabetes on various organs throughout the body.

Well, before we can work on repairing the receptor, we need to understand what's causing the problem in the first place. Again, the medical model suggests that you have just eaten too much sugar and the "cell is full." This is completely false. There can be many reasons why and how the receptors become insulin resistant. The most common are the use of ethanol/alcohol, extreme exercise, hormone imbalances, chemicals in the food we eat, the water we drink, the environment we are living in, and free fatty acids.

Diabetes is a lot like taking your car into a mechanic when the engine won't run. There is gas in the tank, (i.e., glucose), the engine works (i.e., the cell), but the fuel pump (i.e., insulin) will not allow the gas to reach the engine. You don't say the gas is bad for the car or say that less gas is better, and you don't fault the engine; you just repair the fuel pump. This is what we need to be doing for the cell's insulin receptor. So, how do we do that?

When we eat a meal with carbohydrates, carbs will be broken down into glucose and glucose will enter the bloodstream. Insulin will be produced by the pancreas, and its binding to the insulin receptors allows the glucose to enter the cells to make energy. Each cell needs enough energy to perform its function(s). As the cell reaches its energy quota, any remaining unused glucose will be stored in the muscle and in the liver as glycogen (i.e., stored glucose) for use when the body needs it later. When the muscle and the liver can no longer store glycogen, the glucose will be converted to fat. We know that the brain and red blood cells prefer glucose as their primary energy source. That means that the levels of glucose in the bloodstream need to be within in a fairly tight range, normally around 70-100 ng/mL, in order to meet the body's energy demands. The body will make adjustments and compensations to maintain the blood sugar within this range. Glycogen (i.e., stored glucose) can be depleted within eight to twenty-four hours with a healthy liver, and in a far shorter time with an unhealthy liver.

How does the body create the glucose if you don't eat enough calories or if you consistently eat a low carb diet?

We discussed earlier that the body has the ability to convert amino acids into glucose through the process of *gluconeogenesis*, which is the new production of glucose. What are the hormones that regulate this new production? They are the stress hormones, cortisol and adrenaline; remember them? Whenever you're eating a low carb diet or when you're in a fasting state, your body goes into a stress response mode that will break down muscle and even do damage to various organs in order to create glucose; in this process, compounds known as fatty acids will be freed up to burn for energy.[3] Free fatty acids compete with glucose as the cell's source of energy. This phenomenon is known as the *Randle Cycle*, (also known as the glucose-fatty acid cycle) first described in 1963 in the British medical journal *The Lancet*.[4] This cycle takes place predominantly in muscle and fat tissue and controls fuel selection within the cell.[5] When our body uses fat as its primary fuel source, or when it releases fat from the fat cells, this will block the cell's receptors' ability to take in glucose for energy, which will inevitably lead to insulin resistance.

This can make logical sense if you think about it. What is the alarm mechanism that tells your body's physiology to change when there's a famine, and how does it know that you are starving? It is when you start burning fat for fuel. As we mentioned earlier, when your body enters that stress state, it will slow your metabolism in order to allow you to survive longer. It does this by lowering your youth/anti-aging hormones.

By not eating enough calories consistently, by limiting carbs, and by eating more fat, you will inevitably put yourself in an ongoing stressed state, and we have already seen how bad stress is for us, regardless of whether it's short term or long term.

Anyone who has ever tried going "keto," or has tried switching to a low carb diet, is actually trying to achieve a state of ketosis (i.e., burning fat for energy). It takes many hours, or even days, to be able to reach a true ketosis state, and just one meal containing carbs will eliminate ketosis.

When there are a lot of free fatty acids floating around the body, we will see increased inflammatory markers, such as elevated NF-κβ (Nuclear Factor Kappa Beta) and TNF-α (Tumor Necrosis Factor Alpha), which are both inflammatory cytokines.[6] We will talk about inflammation in a separate chapter, but we now know that chronic inflammation is part of most disease processes we are dealing with in society today. Chronic inflammatory diseases include cancer, diabetes, cardiovascular disease, autoimmune diseases like lupus, rheumatoid arthritis, Hashimoto's thyroiditis, and even clinical depression. This type of chronic inflammation can happen not just in obese people, but also in people with no weight problems.

There are a number of several long-distance runners who are lean, and yet, they suffer from chronic inflammation and are also insulin resistant.[7] This is due to their use of FFAs for fuel in long duration exercise such as running marathons. Shorter duration, higher intensity exercises, like running sprints or weight training, are not as likely to contribute to chronic inflammatory processes. One of the hallmarks of aging is the cell losing its ability to turn glucose into energy (i.e., oxidize glucose). One process of converting a substance into energy within the cell is a process referred to as oxidation. The aging cell prefers fat as an energy source in this process because the aging cell has lost its ability to turn glucose into energy. This also happens in Type 2 diabetics, regardless of age. We see this in teenagers who can eat candy and sugary cereals and maintain low blood sugar levels, while an older person eats one bite of dessert and their blood sugar levels go sky-high. The aging cell and the diabetic cell have trouble switching from fat oxidation to glucose oxidation. It should use glucose for energy because, as we mentioned earlier, it's the body's preferred energy source. But it can't.[8]

## Takeaways from Chapter 5

1. Diabetes is an inability to make insulin or an inability for the pancreas to make adequate levels of insulin.

2. Non-insulin-dependent diabetes, (commonly referred to as Type 2) is caused mainly by sedentary lifestyle, chronic stress, and poor diet. It's epidemic in westernized society.

3. Insulin resistance and high blood sugar are symptoms, but not the actual cause, of diabetes. Restricting our carbs/sugar intake is not fixing the problem but is an attempt at damage control.

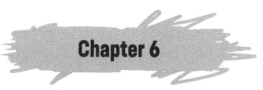

# Chapter 6

# Thyroid Hormones

We talked about the master gland being the hypothalamus, but now we will discuss the master metabolic hormone of the body, which is the thyroid hormone. This is the master metabolic hormone because it dictates how the body utilizes energy. There are several different forms of thyroid hormone; however, we will focus on T4 and T3 (inactive versus active, respectively).

The two main thyroid hormones that we will discuss here, that are actively involved in the bioenergetic model of health, are T4 and T3. The technical name for T4 is *thyroxine*, which is the inactive form of thyroid hormone. The technical name for T3 is *triiodothyronine*, which is the active form of thyroid hormone. Ninety-two percent of what the thyroid releases is the inactive form T4 with only 8% released as T3. T4 travels to the liver and to other body tissues to be converted by the help of enzymes into its active form of T3. Eighty to ninety percent of the inactive hormone T4 is converted in the liver. This is one of the reasons a healthy liver is so incredibly important for energy/metabolism. Any disruption in liver function can cause significant problems in meeting the body's energy needs. As of 2020, up to 50% of Americans are suffering from *non-alcoholic fatty liver disease* (NAFLD). This can impair the function of the liver and can also cause thyroid dysfunction.[1]

In the introduction and throughout this book, we talk about the bioenergetic model of health. To refresh your memory, the bioenergetic model of health focuses on the fact that optimal health requires interdependent energy, function, and structure. This means that if there is enough energy, the cell will function as it is physiologically designed to do and will have enough energy to repair itself as needed. On the other hand, when there is deficient energy, the cell cannot function properly and will even dismantle its own energy generator inside the cell (i.e., *mitochondria*) in order to conserve energy. We can expand this to the whole body, such that when cells are lacking optimal energy, the body is also lacking optimal energy. Then, you'll start to see symptoms like fatigue, weight gain, injury, inability to build muscle, and problems with skin, nails, hair, and digestive issues. You'll also see the body lack enough energy for adequate sex drive and reproduction.

Thyroid hormones are produced by the thyroid gland, which is a butterfly-shaped gland in the front of the neck. Every cell in the body needs active thyroid hormone, T3 (triiodothyronine), in order to function and to do its job.

Remember the hypothalamus and the pituitary glands that we discussed in Chapter 3? It was there that we introduced the feedback system known as the hypothalamic-pituitary-adrenal axis (HPA), which works as a negative feedback system, to regulate the production of thyroid hormones. The thyroid gland plays a pivotal role in this system, as it releases a compound known as *thyrotropin releasing hormone*, (TRH, for short). This system works to respond to the body's energy demands like your thermostat at home works to respond to your home's heating and cooling needs. When there is a need for more thyroid hormone, the hypothalamus-pituitary gland releases more TRH, which signals the thyroid to produce more thyroid hormone. When there is enough of the active thyroid hormone circulating around the bloodstream, this will signal the HPA axis to stop producing TRH. This is an example of a negative feedback system.

There are two main types of thyroid problems that will actively interfere with optimal health. One is the condition of an overactive thyroid, referred to as *hyperthyroidism*, and the other is that of an underactive thyroid, referred to as *hypothyroidism*.

The most common thyroid problem is an underactive thyroid or hypothyroidism. This can be caused from a dysfunction at the level of the hypothalamus or the pituitary gland, but this is actually pretty rare. Hypothyroid dysfunction is generally a failure at the thyroid gland itself and accounts for 95% of hypothyroid cases.

This is one of the most common conditions that we see clinically. A person with hypothyroidism will have one or more of a combination of symptoms, such as fatigue, weight gain, depression, anxiety, thinning hair, brittle nails, lowered sex drive, dry skin, lowered body temperature, and/or constipation.[2] Often, they have seen many healthcare providers to complain of these symptoms, thinking they might be having problems with their thyroid, only to be told that nothing is wrong or their labs look fine. If they are lucky, they might actually get a diagnosis of subclinical hypothyroidism. As treatment, they would generally be given the inactive form of the thyroid hormone, T4 (generic name, *levothyroxine*). This might make their lab results appear more normal, but too often the person would still be experiencing all the symptoms, since the liver/body may not be able to convert the inactive form into the active form, or the active form may not be able to be utilized by the body's cells.

When the primary complaints were fatigue and weight gain, the patient would generally hear their provider telling them to eat less and exercise more in order to lose weight and have more energy. When a person has true hypothyroidism, this would be the worst advice. When a person has a truly underactive thyroid, this would only make things worse. Fixing an underactive thyroid requires much more than dieting and exercise.

In fact, as far back as the 1950s through 1970s, Dr. Broda Barnes, MD, the father of thyroid medicine and one of the leading thyroid experts of the time, recognized and estimated that approximately 40% of women and/or men without symptoms had some form of hypothyroidism.[3] This is still the case today. So, why are subclinical (not detectable by the usual clinical tests) hypothyroid conditions diagnosed so infrequently? The main reason is that modern medicine does not always consider the complicated pathways involved in thyroid hormone production and/or function when screening for or attempting to diagnose an underactive thyroid.

Moreover, and much more problematic, is the fact that these problems are the result of thyroid conditions undetectable by normal clinical testing. Let's look at some of the shortcomings of the labs currently used to assess for adequate thyroid function. The majority of the time, the only lab test that is performed is TSH, which is short for *thyroid stimulating hormone*. This is the pituitary hormone that tells the thyroid what to do. When the body needs more thyroid hormone, the pituitary gland will release TSH in order to stimulate the thyroid to release more thyroid hormone.

We have seen that when the body has enough thyroid hormone, this will feed back to the pituitary to lower the TSH, and, as a result, the thyroid will cut back on its release of thyroid hormones. The confusing part to patients, however, and even perhaps to some medical professionals, is that because this system is working as a negative feedback loop, the TSH value is inverse to the amount of thyroid hormone being released—meaning, a high TSH level is telling us that there is too little thyroid hormone being released (i.e., underactive thyroid or hypothyroid condition). On the other hand, when the TSH level is low, this tells us that there is actually a lot of thyroid hormone being released (i.e., overactive thyroid or hyperthyroid condition).

All of this would be fine, if, most of the time, the problem was actually at the thyroid level, but we know that a primary cause of the symptoms of an underactive thyroid most often occur outside the thyroid, throughout the body at the cellular level. Remember, we said that every cell in the body needs the active thyroid hormone (i.e., T3) in order to function and to do its job, and that 92% of the thyroid hormone released by the thyroid is in the inactive form (i.e., T4).

There are several ways in which these problems occur.

Symptoms of an underactive thyroid can be the result of enzymes not converting the inactive hormone (T4) to its active state (T3). Yet another problem can occur when enzymes are deactivating the active hormone (T3) after its conversion, which will also make the thyroid hormone unusable. In all of these situations, the person's TSH level may appear normal, and the person's thyroid declared healthy and functional, when in reality the body is deficient of useable thyroid hormone (i.e., in an underactive thyroid state).

Another major problem with our current lab testing method is attempting to measure the function of the thyroid gland by TSH level, in which the "normal" range is huge. The normal range is typically anywhere from 0.5-4.5 milli-international units per liter, or mlU\L. This means we're looking at a ten-fold spread from the bottom of the range to the top of the range. If your TSH levels are at the bottom of the healthy range (remember, lower levels imply higher amounts of thyroid hormone), you may have almost ten times the thyroid hormone as a person at the top of the TSH range (where higher levels imply lower amounts of active thyroid hormone).[4] Dr. Barnes actually thought that anyone with a TSH over 1.5 mlU\L of TSH had an underactive thyroid.[5] Many people have TSH levels that are showing in the high range of normal, and their endocrinologist may tell them that they are simply fine, nothing needed, that they can come back in six months and re-test.

Occasionally, the actual thyroid hormones will be tested, most commonly T4. Many doctors are ordering TSH levels routinely that will automatically generate a T4 level, if their TSH levels are out of range. However, if the TSH levels are falling within the lab's "normal" range, usually no further testing will occur. Because T4 is the inactive form of the thyroid hormone and must be converted into the active form of T3 to be able to have its effects on the cell, it is a better indicator of adequate thyroid hormone function than just testing TSH by itself. As we demonstrated above, there are many situations in which enzymes interfere with the conversion of T4 (inactive) into T3 (active) throughout the body. If there is liver dysfunction, the body's ability to convert T4 (inactive) into T3 (active) will be affected. As we mentioned earlier, most notably, this can occur with a condition known as NAFLD (non-alcoholic fatty liver disease) in which the buildup of fat cells in the liver occurs where the cause is not alcohol.[6] It is thought that approximately 25 to 50% of Western societies have this condition, with 25% of those showing normal liver function lab tests.

In a rare case, a doctor will order a T3 measurement. This is actually measuring the active form of thyroid hormone, but it still does not show how the active thyroid hormone is acting at the cell and/or at the receptor site. If lab tests do not show the correct levels, then how do you know if your thyroid is functioning properly? Great question.

Before these types of lab tests, hypothyroidism (i.e., underactive thyroid condition) was diagnosed clinically by patient's reports of symptoms, such as the following:

- fatigue
- weight gain
- injury
- inability to build muscle
- problems with dry skin
- digestive issues, like constipation

- low sex drive
- infertility
- menstrual cycle irregularities
- low testosterone
- depression
- anxiety
- thinning hair
- brittle nails

Research shows that the body temperature of the average person has decreased in recent years. The researchers explain the decrease as a result of "having fewer infections than in previous years."[7] This is the explanation we get from people who do not seem to take into account the complexity of the thyroid's function in energy and metabolism. A more accurate method of determining adequate thyroid function would be by pulse and body temperature. Remember that T4 and T3 are the energy and metabolism hormones. Energy produces heat; this is how we maintain a body temperature of 98.6 degrees Fahrenheit. One of the most common complaints of people with low thyroid is feeling cold all of the time. When other people are warm, a person with an underactive thyroid condition is wearing a sweater, or a person may have the heat on when it is warm outside.

We need to differentiate between *primary hypothyroidism* (happening at the thyroid gland) and *functional hypothyroidism* (occurring at the cellular level throughout the body). Primary hypothyroidism occurs with chronic stress within the gland itself, which leads to lower T4 (inactive) hormone levels and lowered T3 (active) hormone levels. In contrast, when the blood levels of T4 (inactive) and T3 (active) remain normal, but the uptake of T4 (inactive) and/or T3 (active) into the cell is blocked, this is what is referred to as functional hypothyroidism. The TSH levels (thyroid stimulating hormone produced by the pituitary gland) can remain normal in both cases. There are studies that show that stress reduces the cellular uptake of T4 and T3 by anywhere from 50 to 79%, all while the TSH levels remain normal.

An example of functional hypothyroidism is the reduction in thyroid hormones that occurs when you diet. Acute and chronic dieting have been shown to reduce T3 (active) hormone within the cell by up to 50% (chronic dieting is defined as dieting for more than two to three months). Also, when you diet, free fatty acids increase in the bloodstream and are thereby seen as an energy source for the body. When this happens, it causes a huge drop in your resting *basal metabolic rate* (i.e., how many calories you burn at rest), anywhere from 15 to 40%. This is a protective mechanism to reduce energy expenditure in response to actual or perceived starvation. This reduction of metabolism will persist for months to years after the person stops dieting. Individuals who had lost weight in the past showed a significant reduction in metabolism of 25% compared to the same-weight individuals who had not lost weight from dieting. This would mean that the person who has not dieted may burn up to six hundred more calories than someone who lost weight through dieting. People often think that a person is failing at a diet because they are eating too much; in reality, they can eat less than normal and still continue to put on weight. We will discuss this in detail in the section on nutrition/diet.[8]

We have discussed previously the negative effects of insulin resistance. Interestingly, there is a connection between insulin resistance and the thyroid. With insulin resistance, there happens to be a reduction in active thyroid conversion (T4 converted to T3) and a reduction in T3 concentration within the cell. Increased insulin also suppresses TSH levels from the pituitary, which will mean that the thyroid won't know to make more thyroid hormone when needed.

The less frequent thyroid problem is hyperthyroidism, where the thyroid produces more hormone than the body needs. There are three main causes of this condition, but for our purposes here, we will be talking predominantly about the autoimmune condition called *Grave's disease*. As with all autoimmune conditions, the body's immune system is attacking itself. In this case, the body's immune system is attacking the thyroid gland and associated tissues. Thyroid hormone will spill out of the gland as it is being destroyed, causing significant excess of thyroid hormone circulating throughout the body. This can be a life-threatening disease if left untreated. One of the classic symptoms of hyperthyroidism is bulging of the eyes, a condition that the comedian Marty Feldman was known for.

Here are some of the other symptoms of hyperthyroidism:
- excessive sweating

- heat intolerance
- frequent bowel movements
- tremors
- nervousness
- anxiety
- rapid heart rate, palpitations, irregular heart rate
- weight loss
- fatigue
- weakness
- irregular and light menstrual cycles
- fine/brittle hair
- thinning skin
- insomnia

One treatment for hyperthyroidism is a medication that blocks the conversion of T4 hormone (inactive) to T3 (active), lowering levels of the active thyroid hormone in the bloodstream. However, the current treatment protocol for hyperthyroidism is not medication: it is either surgical removal of the thyroid gland or treatment of the gland with radioactive iodine. The latter will cause the destruction of the thyroid gland. Surgical removal and radioactive treatment with iodine will leave a person with a low thyroid condition forever, requiring that a person be given thyroid medication for the rest of their life.

An important thyroid disruptor is the presence of environmental toxins, also known as *persistent organic pollutants* (POP). These include pollutants such as PCBs, pesticides, plastics, and phthalates. These can be found in foods we eat, the water we drink, our skin care products, our cookware, and food containers, to name a few sources. They are found everywhere. These types of toxins have been shown to block thyroid hormones' entry into the cell and create lower levels of thyroid hormones throughout the body.[9]

Other factors that can influence thyroid hormone levels are deficiencies of nutrients such as iodine, selenium, zinc, and/or certain amino acids from proteins.

The main takeaway from this chapter is that blood tests that determine thyroid levels and thyroid function are relatively unreliable when it comes to identifying true hypothyroid or hyperthyroid conditions. If you have been told that your thyroid levels are normal, yet you are still suffering with symptoms, there's a strong possibility that your thyroid is having problems, regardless of what your clinical lab levels suggest.

Our objective is to restore your thyroid to its proper function and balance out the appropriate levels of thyroid hormones. We will go into how to work with diet, supplementation, and lifestyle changes to provide increased energy and optimal metabolism. This will allow you to get back to the energy levels and metabolism of your youth. Just imagine if you were able to speed up your metabolism—the metabolism you had when you were younger, without starving yourself in order to maintain your weight. Keep reading.

Although other anti-aging hormones play a pivotal role in our optimal health, for the subject matter at hand, we will be saving these for another time. Working to optimize the estrogen/progesterone balance, blood sugar regulation, and thyroid function will go a long way to improving our overall health. Now, let's visit the subject of inflammation—something we hear a lot about these days and one of our biggest risk factors for increased mortality and a shortened life span.

---

## Takeaways from Chapter 6

1. Acute or chronic dieting (more than two to three months) can reduce active thyroid hormone levels by up to 50%. The thyroid gland is our main metabolism center.

2. There are several different forms of thyroid hormone; we are focusing on the inactive form T4 and the active form T3.

3. Current lab testing does not allow us to know where most of the problems are occurring when our thyroid is underactive. A more accurate measurement is heart rate and body temperature.

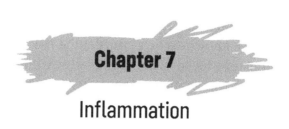

# Chapter 7

# Inflammation

Inflammation and stress go hand in hand. We have discussed the negative effects of stress, looking at various biochemical systems and hormones in the body that help and hinder optimal health. Now we will look at the negative effects of inflammation. Chronic inflammation is a silent killer. Inflammation has recently been recognized as the most significant contributor to increased mortality in the modern world. In one particular analysis, inflammation-related deaths were behind more than 280 causes of death in 195 countries and territories, from 1980– 2017.[1] This is profound. Diseases included in the analysis were heart disease, stroke, cancer, diabetes, autoimmune conditions, chronic kidney disease, non-alcoholic fatty liver disease (NAFLD), and neurodegenerative conditions.[2] Inflammation has also been recognized more recently as a major factor in cognitive disorders such as dementia, depression, bipolar disorder, schizophrenia, developmental disabilities, and anxiety.

Unfortunately, inflammation is a confusing and conflicted topic. It can be both the cause and the effect of poor health, dysfunction, and disease. And for many people, when they are seeing their health care professional, it's often not specifically addressed. As with the stress response, there is an acute stage and a chronic stage of inflammatory response. Most of the health problems related to westernized society today arise from ongoing and/or chronic inflammatory processes.[3]

## Covid-19 and Inflammation: Cause and Effect

Highlighting the deadly and devastating impact of inflammation, we can see how COVID-19 has crippled the US economy, unlike any flu epidemic in recent years. In the early days of the pandemic, in an attempt to better understand the virus, limit the mortality rate, and protect those known to be at substantial risk, the government imposed mandatory lockdowns, during which the US suffered an unemployment rate at its highest since the Great Depression in the 1920s.[4] Although we have been in a global pandemic, the American lifestyle has contributed significantly to the case counts and deaths in the US. Unfortunately, this outbreak has exposed the disparities in our society caused by poverty and lack of access to healthcare. Our way of eating, our workaholic society, and our overly sedentary lifestyle have produced an epidemic of co-morbidities and other health conditions that greatly enhance inflammation. Diabetes, chronic heart disease, chronic lung disease, and autoimmune diseases/conditions are among the most prevalent conditions related to chronic inflammation, and, interestingly enough, these four conditions increase mortality in COVID-19 by up to twelve times.

Even though many cases and deaths from COVID-19 have been reported by the news media, it is still not the highest cause of death in this country; cancer and heart disease hold that position. Many of the most prevalent cancers are related to lifestyle, stress, and diet. This has been shown throughout the literature repeatedly for the past five to ten years; however, little has changed. It would be helpful for us to learn some significant lessons from this information—to produce significant advances in treating, managing, and minimizing chronic inflammatory conditions, helping all Americans to work toward a goal of access to healthcare and, thus, optimal health and wellness.[5]

Now, let's define what inflammation is. Inflammation is simply an immune system response to some type of irritant. The irritant can be from a foreign invader such as bacteria, a virus, or a parasite. It can also be a response to an any type of injury such as a sprained ankle or car accident, or any type of trauma. It can be a response to chemical/toxin exposure. It can be a response to radiation, or it can be an allergic response.

When you have an inflammatory response, many different immune cells are involved.[6] These immune cells are generated through an elaborate system involving the bone marrow, the spleen, and the thymus gland. The immune cells will release chemicals, primarily *histamine* and *bradykinin*, which will signal the need to mount a defense. Most people know histamine from taking antihistamine medication for seasonal allergies or rashes like poison ivy. Both histamine and bradykinin cause the blood vessels to *vasodilate*, which means the blood vessels expand to bring more blood flow and, therefore, more immune cells into the area. Both are also nerve irritants that lead to pain. When you have acute inflammation, there are five cardinal signs: swelling, redness, heat, pain, and loss of function. These cardinal signs are part of the body's protective system that limits the mobility of the area, as in the case of a sprained ankle or other injury. However, often, as with a systemic infection, some of the inflammatory symptoms will be "silent," presenting with primarily nondescript symptoms such as fatigue, fever, or a just a feeling of being unwell.

There are many other types of mediators—white blood cells (leukocytes), T cells, and cytokines that come to the damaged area to clean up debris from the injury or fight off the invader(s). The following are conditions that can cause acute inflammation:

- bacteria
- virus
- parasite
- injury

So, that is the acute inflammatory response, but the more detrimental phase—and the one that we are more concerned about—is chronic inflammation, the kind that can last for weeks, months, and even years. Chronic inflammation can follow an acute phase or can occur for what seems to be no apparent reason without any known acute injury or insult.

Chronic inflammation has both tissue repair and tissue destruction happening simultaneously. This, in turn, leads to the formation of new blood vessels and fibrosis, (i.e., scarring). Here are some of the causes of chronic inflammation:

- chronic infections from bacteria/viruses (Lyme disease, tuberculosis, or hepatitis C)
- allergies

- food intolerances
- pollutants
- toxins
- autoimmune conditions
- parasites
- gastrointestinal dysfunction
- even supplements, like omega-6

Here are some examples of diseases that are associated with chronic inflammation:

- infections like tuberculosis caused by bacteria, which leads to fibrosis and scarring of the lungs
- hepatitis C caused by a virus that can lead to cirrhosis of the liver and scarring of the liver from advanced fibrosis
- bladder infections like cystitis—these are usually caused by bacteria and can lead to scarring in the bladder
- toxins, such as asbestos and adulterants from cigarettes/vaping can lead to mesothelioma, inflammatory lung diseases such as *Chronic Obstructive Pulmonary Disease* (COPD), and lipoid pneumonia

*Systemic inflammation*, meaning inflammation throughout the entire body, can lead to diseases such as coronary artery disease, heart attacks, and stroke.

Autoimmune conditions occur when the immune system turns on itself and attacks certain cells of the body. There are many autoimmune conditions; examples of a few are the following:

- Hashimoto thyroiditis
- lupus
- osteoarthritis
- rheumatoid arthritis
- psoriasis
- multiple sclerosis

So, as we demonstrated above, chronic inflammation can be both the result of an ongoing condition(s), as well as the cause of dysfunction/disease. In fact, low-grade inflammation is a significant contributor to age-related comorbidity and mortality. This process has been coined *inflammaging*.[7]

Inflammaging is the natural tendency toward more inflammation as we age. Chronic inflammation has been shown to develop with advanced age, a result of weight gain, poor diet, poor sleep, and chronic stress. Other contributors to inflammaging are persistent viral infections, increased intestinal permeability, and/or autoimmune conditions.[8] If the immune system is chronically overactive, this can lead to Type 2 diabetes, clinical depression, and even Alzheimer's disease.[9]

One of the major results of inflammation is that it activates the stress response. Remember that cortisol is the body's natural anti-inflammatory hormone, so when there is any inflammation, especially chronic inflammation, the body stays in a "fight or flight mode." In fact, cortisol is such a powerful anti-inflammatory that healthcare providers commonly use the steroid medication cortisone on the skin or prednisone orally to treat inflammatory conditions. These medications were developed to mimic the body's natural anti-inflammatory, cortisol. When cortisol levels remain high for any prolonged length of time, the immune system response is suppressed.

If you remember what we discussed in the chapter about cortisol, we talked about cortisol causing destruction of the thymus gland. The thymus gland plays a significant role in the immune system, and any destruction of the thymus gland will compromise the body's ability to mount an adequate immune system response.

As you will recall, one of the hallmarks of cortisol is storing visceral fat. Visceral fat in turn has shown to increase levels of inflammatory markers. It appears that numerous inflammatory mediators are produced and excreted from fat tissue.

Chronic inflammation is a feature of the condition known as *metabolic syndrome*, which is a collection of symptoms of increased blood pressure, increased blood sugar, fat around the waist, and increased cholesterol or *triglyceride* levels. This syndrome raises the risk of cardiac disease, stroke, and diabetes. Metabolic syndrome has become increasingly common. Up to a third of the population of the United States has metabolic syndrome, high blood pressure, increased abdominal girth, high triglyceride levels, and increased body mass index (BMI).

Local inflammation within fat tissue may be the cause for systemic insulin resistance and systemic inflammation, which are two of the key factors causing metabolic syndrome. Chronic inflammation can also be a cause of cancer. In 1863, the German scientist Rudolf Virchow was one of the first to write about observing cancer in places where there was chronic inflammation. Recent data has shown that chronic inflammation is critical in the formation and progression of tumor formation.[10] It has become clear that the microenvironment in the tissues plays an important part in tumor formation. Many cancers start at the sites of chronic irritation and/or sites of infection where inflammation is occurring.

Chronic inflammatory conditions such as pancreatitis, colitis, Crohn's disease, and hepatitis B and C are linked to a greater risk of pancreatic, colon, and liver cancers, respectively. Also, chronic infections with *H. pylori* can lead to stomach cancer. HPV can lead to cervical cancer.[11]

One of the most important causes of inflammation, though, is from some of the foods we eat. This can be from a certain type of fat that is the precursor to inflammatory chemicals (i.e., omega-6 is precursor to arachidonic acid, which is precursor to leukotrienes, COX-2 compounds).[12] Nitrites, salts, or esters of nitrous acid found in smoked foods increase the risk of colon cancer.[13] We will go into great detail in the diet section of the book. A major contributor of systemic inflammation is the gastrointestinal tract: the digestion of certain foods we eat releases toxins into the bloodstream. We will cover this in the next chapter about GI function.

The main takeaway about inflammation is that chronic inflammation has a detrimental effect on the body, and its symptoms can often be silent. We need to know how to minimize the risks of chronic inflammation in order to feel our best and obtain optimal health as we age. We will show you how to control inflammation in Part Three of this book. Stay tuned.

## Takeaways from Chapter 7

1. Chronic inflammation is endemic in our society and is a silent killer; it's behind many of the underlying health conditions we experience today.

2. Inflammaging is the natural tendency toward more inflammation as we age.

3. One of the most important causes of inflammation is from some of the foods we eat.

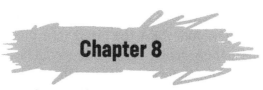

# Chapter 8

## Gastrointestinal Tract

Maybe one of the most important keys to our optimal health is a healthy gastrointestinal (GI) tract. Most people rarely think of their gastrointestinal tract in terms of how healthy they are or how well their immune system is functioning. We do not usually think about it until we have some type of dysfunction like heartburn, reflux, bloating, gas, or other bowel problems such as constipation and/or diarrhea. Then we reach for some type of medication to stop the symptoms, not even thinking of what the underlying problems are or why they are happening. We have heard people say that they don't have issues with their digestion because they take Nexium (i.e., proton-pump inhibitor) every day. When asking them what happens if they don't take it, they say they have indigestion or they say they can't sleep because they can't "lay flat." Our thought for them, and even for you, is that wouldn't it be better to find out why there is a problem, fix the problem, and avoid all the side effects of medications?

This is why we're writing this book: we're writing it for you, for the everyday American. The example just given—and there are many more where that came from—is just a microcosm of how we have come to look at our health. If there is a problem, we have the mindset of just taking a pill to "fix" the symptoms, instead of truly identifying what the problem is at a functional level and then taking the steps necessary to address the issue(s).

Before we get into how particular GI problems have an effect on our overall health, it's important to understand some basic anatomy and the overall general function of the GI tract. The GI tract starts at your mouth and ends at the outlet of the rectum (anus). First, we have the mouth, the first part of digestion. Its role is to process the food into smaller pieces. When you chew, it releases enzymes to start the digestive process. It's important to chew your food well so the stomach doesn't have to work as hard in digesting and liquefying the food. The more you can chew your food, the better your digestion will be. The teeth also play an important part in your overall health. If there is any periodontal disease or infection of the teeth and gums, this can easily turn into systemic inflammation and disease throughout the rest of the body. Recent research shows that infections of the teeth and gums are known to cause heart disease.[1]

## Stomach

Once the food passes from the mouth to the stomach, the stomach will basically liquefy the food into what is called *chyme* (basically, mush). Chyme is created by active movements of the stomach that churn and mix the food with hydrochloric acid and digestive enzymes like pepsin. The stomach releases *hydrochloric acid* (HCl) to digest protein, especially meat. The pH of the stomach should be nearly the most acidic place on the planet. Not only is it important for digesting meat, but it is also highly proactive in killing off bacteria, viruses, and/or parasites to prevent them from getting into the body.

When you don't have enough hydrochloric acid, your food will not digest well. It will start to ferment in the stomach, and a lot like making wine, will create $CO_2$ gas, which, in turn, will cause bloating, belching, and indigestion. So, interestingly, the current medical model suggests, "Let's stop the acid; then you won't get the bloating from the build-up of gas." Why is this a problem? Well, first, the food sits in the stomach and doesn't digest well before being moved on further through the digestive tract. Second, the hydrochloric acid is there to kill bacteria, viruses, and parasites, so when there is not enough stomach acid, you become much more susceptible to invasive pathogens. And third, you need the stomach to be acidic in order to better absorb calcium, magnesium, and other minerals.

A better question would be, "Why would a person not make enough stomach acid in the first place?" The most common reasons are from the stress response, from a nutritional deficiency, or from a dietary deficiency. We can see an example of a dietary deficiency in people who eat a vegetarian or vegan diet. In both cases, the body will decrease its production of HCl since no digestion of meat is required.

There are problems when you don't have enough HCl, but what happens when you have too much? Actually, the only time that too much HCl in the stomach is a problem is when you have an ulcer, which is an irritation and erosion of the stomach lining. Ulcers can be a serious medical problem, as this irritation and erosion can lead to internal bleeding and require emergency medical attention. An ulcer is most often caused by either a bacterial infection from *H. pylori* (helicobacter pylori) or from medication, usually non-steroidal anti-inflammatory medications (also known as NSAIDS, i.e., aspirin, ibuprofen, Aleve). One of the most commonly prescribed medications for ulcers is antacid medication. Is there ever a time to use an antacid? Yes, when there is an ulcer. Antacid medication is used to decrease the acid production in the stomach in order to help the stomach lining heal. These medications, however, are never meant to be long-term therapies.

## Gallbladder

The gallbladder is a small organ located beneath the liver. The gallbladder releases bile into the first section of the small intestine immediately adjacent to the stomach (*duodenum*). Bile is produced in the liver and stored in the gallbladder. Bile is a fat *emulsifier*, which means it breaks up fat. Think of it like dishwashing soap: if you try to wash a greasy pan with just water, the fat lays on top of the water, but, if you add dish soap, it breaks up the grease. Why is it so important to emulsify fat? Because without emulsifying fat, you risk becoming deficient in vitamins that are fat soluble (namely, vitamins A, D, E, K). We will talk more about the fat-soluble vitamins in the nutrition part of this book.

Gallbladder issues are fairly common. The gallbladder can either be filled with gallstones that form from undissolved cholesterol that has crystallized with bile, or the undissolved cholesterol can become thick and sludge-like. When either of these things happen, a person can begin to have pronounced pain in the right side of their abdomen. A person can even feel like they are having a heart attack, when what's actually happening is a "gallbladder attack." The main medical treatment is to remove the gallbladder. If you are one of the unfortunate people who have had your gallbladder removed, you will have difficulty digesting fatty meals. This can be resolved by taking a bile salts supplement with every meal in order to aid in the digestion of fats. A much better approach to any problem in the gallbladder is to thin the bile and/or dissolve the stones so that the gallbladder can work the way it should. The only exception to this would be if a stone becomes lodged in the bile duct, which then becomes a true medical emergency. However, this condition is a fairly rare occurrence. Of the many people who have come to our offices without their gallbladder, none have ever been recommended for alternative treatment. So, as a result of living without a gallbladder, they suffer from chronic gas and bowel issues that require a supplement with every meal.

## Small Intestine

Once the food is made into chyme in the stomach, it travels to the small intestine. The first part of the small intestine, as mentioned above, is known as the duodenum, which is adjacent to the stomach and begins where the stomach ends. The stomach empties its contents into the duodenum, usually about four to five hours after eating. The duodenum is where the gallbladder releases bile. Bile is needed here, as this is the place where fat digestion begins in the digestive tract. Because of the duodenum's proximity to the stomach, it is a common place for ulcers, usually due to H. pylori and/or chronic use of medications like ibuprofen, Aleve, or other NSAIDs, as noted above. Just like in the stomach, this infection and/or these medications will erode the lining of the duodenal wall.

The small intestine, specifically the duodenum, is also the site for release of several digestive enzymes from the pancreas—*amylase*, *trypsin*, and *lipase*—that are produced in the pancreas and are responsible for the digestion of proteins, carbohydrates, and fats. Another common cause for GI dysfunction is a lack of digestive enzymes. If there is dysfunction in the pancreas, the production of pancreatic enzymes will decrease, which will greatly affect the ability of the small intestine to breakdown the carbohydrates, proteins, and fats into basic nutrients for absorption. In addition, the duodenum releases bicarbonate to decrease the acidity of the chyme before it continues throughout the rest of the digestive tract. The remainder of the small intestine digests and absorbs a majority of the nutrients from the food that's been eaten. Most malabsorption problems occur in the small intestine, since the main function of the small intestine is to absorb nutrients and minerals from the digested food before it reaches the large intestine.

A serious GI condition that can cause significant inflammation throughout the entire body often begins in the small intestine, but can occur anywhere in the digestive tract. This is a condition known as *Crohn's disease*, which is one form of inflammatory bowel disease. Some of the symptoms are persistent diarrhea, rectal bleeding, urgent need for bowel movement, abdominal pain, incomplete bowel evacuation, constipation, loss of appetite, weight loss, and fatigue. The cause of Crohn's disease is unknown, but many doctors suspect that it is related to a food intolerance similar to celiac disease, which is known to be caused from a gluten intolerance. Crohn's disease may be caused by a variety of other foods including gluten or by other toxins, such as environmental toxins or food additives. The non-medical treatment for Crohn's disease is to find and identify the foods/toxins that are causative and that are contributing to the underlying inflammatory response.

*Celiac disease* is another inflammatory bowel disease caused by a gluten intolerance. It creates inflammation of the small intestine, leading to malabsorption of nutrients. The symptoms include abdominal pain, gas, bloating, diarrhea, fatigue, and weight loss.

Gluten is a protein found in wheat, rye, barley, and, sometimes, oats. It is the substance that makes dough sticky. We'll talk more about gluten in the next section on dieting.

There is also non-celiac gluten intolerance, which is a less severe type of intolerance. It creates many of the same symptoms, as well as other systemic symptoms including fatigue, depression, anxiety, brain fog, skin problems, and joint pain. There is still not a consensus from the medical community on what the occurrence rate is for non-celiac gluten intolerance.[2]

Another serious and fairly common condition that affects the small intestine is *small intestinal bacterial overgrowth* (SIBO). The GI tract is host to a large number of bacteria that are necessary and essential for optimal health and a strong immune system. The majority of these bacteria will be found in the large intestine (i.e., the colon). Although the small intestine should ideally be free of bacteria, fungus, and/or parasites, if there is an overgrowth of bacteria in the large intestine, the bacteria can and will migrate up into the small intestine. When this happens, we refer to this condition as SIBO. It causes many problems both with digestion and with the body's immune system, creating significant inflammation and subsequent long-term health conditions that are not likely to get easily diagnosed by a visit to your primary care provider (PCP) or even gastrointestinal specialist.

A type of infection that can occur in the small intestine and that causes systemic disease is *candidiasis*.[3] You may have heard of someone having a "yeast infection" (i.e., candidiasis). This is caused by a fungus, *Candida albicans* (*C. albicans* or *Candida*). This fungus can take up residence in different parts of the body such as the small intestine and can also cause an array of health problems. Yeast infections of the skin, nails, and vagina can be common with people with suppressed immune systems. Problems in the small intestine can suppress the immune system.

One thought is that low-carb diets can lead to a more aggressive form of systemic candidiasis, namely *invasive candidiasis*. This invasive candidiasis can be a profoundly serious infection that enters the bloodstream and travels to the heart, brain, eyes, bones, skin, and other parts of the body. It is thought that this condition can occur when no food source is available for the *C. albicans* in the large intestine, and it then migrates upward through the GI tract, looking for a more adequate food source.

## Large Intestine (Colon) and Intestinal Bacteria

Once food has traveled through the small intestine and the nutrients have been absorbed, what's left reaches the large intestine, also referred to as the colon. The large intestine is the site in the digestive tract where water, minerals, and electrolytes are resorbed by the body. Most carbohydrates, such as sugar and fruits, are absorbed quickly in the small intestine, but fiber and starches make it to the colon largely undigested. (Of note, starches are molecules made up of long chains of sugars, specifically glucose.) Although the small intestine is designed to be bacteria-free, the colon has bacteria that will help digest the food waste from the rest of the digestive tract. This is usually material that is indigestible by the body's own digestive mechanisms (i.e., fiber and starches). We are trained to think that bacteria are bad and unwanted, but beneficial bacteria do exist. These bacteria, for our purposes, will be referred to as "good bacteria." They will digest the leftover food waste by means of a fermentation process. The "good" bacteria also produce some vitamins like vitamin B12 and vitamin K.

The large intestine is home to over seven hundred types of bacteria, good and bad; a healthy number can be as many as one hundred trillion organisms. To put that in perspective, you have more bacteria in your GI tract than you have cells in your body. The bottom line: there is substantially less of us and substantially more of them!

This collection of bacteria is often referred to as the microbiome. The microbiome plays a huge role in our health. In fact, this is one of the most important points in this book, namely, that your optimal health is dependent on the health of your GI tract, especially your colon. Research shows that people that are still hunter-gatherers (i.e., indigenous peoples) and people living in non-industrialized countries have a much healthier microbiome. They have a much more diverse collection of bacteria compared to those of us living in westernized countries, with the US population having the least diverse microbiome.

Researchers have found they can determine with great accuracy whether a person is lean or obese by sequencing the microbiome genes. There is a 57% accuracy when looking at the person's genes versus a 90% accuracy when looking at their microbiome genes.[4]

Many studies on mice show that taking the microbiome of a fat mouse and transplanting it into a skinny mouse leads to the skinny mouse becoming morbidly obese. They also found the opposite, that when the microbiome of a skinny mouse is transplanted into a fat mouse, the fat mouse will become skinny.[5]

Even more interesting, the same can be said for transplanting a human microbiome into mice. You will see exactly the same results, that is, a skinny person's microbiome will make a fat mouse skinny, whereas a fat person's microbiome will make a skinny mouse fat.

Researchers have just recently started experiments with weight loss on human-to-human fecal microbiome transplants.[6] But there have been human studies of *fecal microbiome transplants* (FMT) in cases of recurrent *Clostridium difficile* (*C. difficile*), which is well-known to cause severe and life-threatening diarrhea. With the transplant, researchers have seen a 90% cure rate. FMT has also been performed for Crohn's disease with some success, showing rates of remission of up to 44%.[7]

How does the microbiome develop? It starts from the very beginning of our life. Our gut microbiome is populated from our mother as we leave the birth canal. Studies show that babies that are delivered by C-section do not have the same microbiome as children delivered by natural birth.[8] The following is according to Dr. Trevor Lawley, reviewing a UK study published in *Nature*:

> Babies born by C-section lacked strains of commensal bacteria—those typically found in healthy individuals—whereas these bacteria made up most of the gut community of vaginally delivered infants. Instead, the guts of C-section babies were dominated by opportunistic bacteria such as *Enterococcus* and *Klebsiella*, which circulate in hospitals.

"The difference was so stark," Lawley says, that "[we] could take a sample from a child and tell you with a high-level certainty how they were born."[9]

Though it is still not clear how this difference in bacterial colonization from vaginal birth to C-section may affect development or long-term health, there are some researchers who state that these effects normalize over time. How that happens is not clearly understood.[10]

Now, let's look at what causes poor intestinal health, mainly involving the large intestine. We start to have significant health problems when the large intestine begins to house more detrimental bacteria (i.e., "bad" bacteria). The "good" bacteria help digest food and support the health of the intestinal lining by producing a mucus-like substance (like the slimy coating you can find on okra). This substance acts like a barrier to protect the intestinal lining and to keep out foreign invaders—such as the bacteria that live in the intestine, or any bacteria, virus, or parasite that we ingest. When we think about "good" bacteria and "bad" bacteria, we can think of them as two opposing armies. The "good" bacteria keep the "bad" bacteria in check and the numbers low. Problems arise when this gets out of balance and the "bad" bacteria outnumber the "good" bacteria. "Bad" bacteria produce a byproduct called *endotoxin*. Endotoxin is also referred to as *lipopolysaccharide* (LPS)—"lipo" meaning fat, "poly" meaning many, and "saccharide" meaning sugar. Endotoxin (LPS) is toxic, hence its name, endotoxin ("toxin within"). We will talk about endotoxin in the next chapter.

Perhaps one of the most common ways to poor intestinal health is through the use of broad-spectrum antibiotics, taken in high doses for short durations. Though an antibiotic may be necessary to fight some types of infections in the body, such as strep throat, sinus, or ear infections, many times, healthcare providers will prescribe them without necessarily confirming that there is an actual bacterial infection for which an antibiotic is actually needed. This type of indiscriminate antibiotic use kills not only the "bad" bacteria but also the "good" bacteria. Sometimes, after a round of antibiotics, even as short as three to five days, you can develop an overgrowth of "bad" bacteria and/or yeast.

After a course of antibiotics, a person may develop a serious and life-threatening infection from overgrowth of *C. difficile*, bacteria that we all have in our large intestine. Without the "good" bacteria to control it, *C. difficile* will grow out of control and a person will start to develop constant and profound, even life-threatening, diarrhea—up to twenty times per day.

In addition, after a round of antibiotics, a person may also develop an overgrowth of yeast, *Candida albicans*, in the large intestine. *Candida albicans* is a normal inhabitant of the large intestine. It contributes to conditions like thrush or recurrent vaginal yeast infections, both of which can occur after finishing an antibiotic therapy regimen. The problem occurs when it becomes invasive, meaning it migrates from the large intestine to other parts of the body, as noted above. This invasive action happens when the yeast is no longer getting the food that it needs. Migration can also occur when people go on "low carb" diets or are eating extremely low-calorie diets. Simply another reason to eat adequate carbs and avoid ketogenic diets.

It's interesting to note that many of the animals used in the meat industry are given antibiotics in their feed to prevent infections due to the unsanitary and poor conditions in which the animals are raised. These antibiotics will be in the meat when we eat it, so that means that many people buying and consuming these products are absorbing low-dose antibiotics on a daily basis. Is there a time for antibiotics? Yes, of course, but only when necessary. Conversely, there is some current research that shows antibiotics have also been used successfully to treat an overgrowth of "bad" bacteria. There are even some studies that show successful treatment of Crohn's disease and IBS with low-dose, longer-term courses of antibiotics targeting a class of bacteria known as Gram-negative bacteria.

Antibiotics work to eliminate and destroy bacteria, but a healthy intestinal tract needs healthy bacteria. This is how *probiotics* came to be so popular. Probiotics are supplements that have been manufactured with live bacteria, the kind of "good" bacteria meant to recolonize the intestinal tract to provide a healthier microbiome. They are the latest and greatest supplements in the health world, but are they really what is needed? The promise is that you can take a few probiotic pills and have a healthy gastrointestinal tract. This sounds great, but it doesn't really work as planned. Studies show that the bacteria in probiotic supplements only survive in the gut for a short time, not long enough to be of any significant benefit in the long term.

Secondly, if you have healthy stomach acid production and the pH of the stomach is acidic, as it should be, the stomach acid will destroy bacteria, viruses, and/or parasites in the food we digest. This means that most, if not all, the probiotic bacteria would be destroyed.[11]

Thirdly, there is still debate as to which type(s) of bacteria used in probiotics are the most beneficial, since there are hundreds to thousands of different bacteria within the digestive tract. Remember, healthier microbiomes are the ones with the most diversity.

Lastly, and most importantly, a person that is inclined to take a probiotic is probably having some type of gastrointestinal dysfunction. If the digestion is slow and the probiotic does make it through the stomach, it will most likely repopulate the small intestine with bacteria, instead of the colon. This can be a big problem since the small intestine should be bacteria-free. Therefore, taking a probiotic may create self-inflicted small intestinal bowel overgrowth and can make any digestive problem much worse.

There are a few major events that can happen in the large intestine that have catastrophic consequences on your health when they do happen, and they usually happen simultaneously. The first problem is when the wall of the large intestine becomes inflamed. This can occur as a result of a pathogen such as a bacteria, fungus, virus, or parasite. It can also occur from certain foods that we eat. When a person has a food intolerance, this can cause inflammation of the large intestinal wall. Irritation of the large intestinal wall can also result from eating one of the foods that contains inflammatory substances like lectins and/or gluten. We will go into greater detail about food intolerances and inflammatory foods in Parts Two and Three of this book.

Alcohol can also create small and large intestinal inflammation. Stress and maintaining a chronic stress response will also lead to inflammation throughout the body, especially in the digestive tract.

Another major digestive issue that causes significant systemic health problems occurs when toxic substances leak out of the small or large intestines and into the bloodstream.[12] Normally, the intestinal wall only lets extremely small particles of nutrients through to the bloodstream, but as the intestinal wall becomes irritated and inflamed, the openings, called tight junctions, become larger and larger. As a result, larger and larger particles that would normally not be able to pass through are now able to travel through the intestinal wall lining and enter the bloodstream. You will often hear this referred to as "leaky gut." Since these particles are not supposed to be in the bloodstream, the body sees them as foreign invaders and mounts an immune system response, which in turn creates active systemic inflammation throughout the body, just like when you get a bacterial infection such as strep throat.

The body sees the *Streptococcal* bacteria as a foreign invader and mounts an aggressive immune response with all the white blood cells, cytokines, and other immune cells, which create inflammation. This is exactly what happens when any bacteria from the GI tract, "good" or "bad," makes its way into the bloodstream.[13] To make matters worse, molecules of undigested food can also pass through the lining, creating more inflammation and causing even more bacteria to get through, which can also lead to food intolerances and/or food allergies. This can continue in a vicious cycle.

If the unending immune response and the ongoing inflammation aren't bad enough, these bacteria will travel through the bloodstream and migrate to different tissues and organs of the body. Once this happens, it can create conditions in which the body will begin to see its own tissue and/or its own organs as a foreign invader and attack and destroy them with its own immune system. When these bacteria travel to organs such as the pancreas, for example, the immune system will mistakenly attack the cells of the pancreas while it tries to kill the bacteria. As it is killing the bacteria, it is simultaneously destroying the pancreas. This is the basis of an autoimmune disease—i.e., the body's immune system turning on itself and destroying its own cells. The cause of autoimmunity is not always well understood, but recent research suggests that bacteria from the GI tract are a major cause of many autoimmune conditions and even many cancers that we see today. Studies have shown that when the GI bacteria migrate from the intestine to the pancreas, for example, this can be a contributing factor in developing pancreatic cancer. These types of cancers have been successfully treated with antibiotics by killing off the bacteria.[14]

## The Liver

The liver is the main filtration organ of the body. Its function is to filter blood from the digestive tract and the rest of the body. The liver filters toxins and medications. It produces bile acids to break down fats, eliminates excess hormones, converts inactive thyroid hormones into active forms, and stores glucose in the form of glycogen.

Some practitioners say that every patient is a liver case because it plays such an important role in our health. One example is the connection between the intestinal bacteria and the liver. A "leaky gut" allows for translocation of bacteria to the liver through the gut-liver axis. This can lead to many chronic liver diseases, such as non-alcoholic fatty liver disease, liver cirrhosis, immune-mediated liver disease, and even liver cancer.[15]

## Takeaways from Chapter 8

1.  One of the keys to our optimal health is having a healthy GI tract; it plays a vital part in having a healthy immune system.

2.  Too often, antacids, OTC, and/or prescribed medications mask symptoms without solving the underlying problem(s).

3.  Having a healthy gut microbiome—more "good" bacteria than "bad" bacteria—is vital to overall good health.

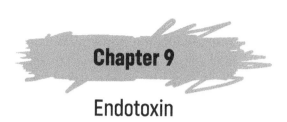

# Chapter 9

## Endotoxin

In the last chapter, we talked about the major players in the GI tract: the stomach, the gallbladder, the small intestine, and the large intestine. So, a quick review of what you have already learned. The small intestine is where most of the nutrients, proteins, carbs, and fats are absorbed into the body. It should be free of bacteria. We discussed a condition called SIBO (small intestinal bowel overgrowth), an overgrowth of bacteria in the large intestine migrating up and into the small intestine. Another common way to develop SIBO is through the use of probiotics.

Now we want to go back to our focus on the large intestine, where most of the problems with "bad" bacteria start. When we talk about inflammation, we need to discuss one very important inhabitant of the GI tract. This is possibly one of the biggest factors in establishing optimal health. We want to delve a little deeper into this so that you understand it completely since your overall health depends on it. This may sound overly dramatic, but plain and simple, if your GI tract is not healthy, you are not healthy.

So, now we'll talk about endotoxin. Though we are separating intestinal bacteria and endotoxin, they are interrelated since the intestinal "bad" bacteria are the usual source of endotoxin. "Good" and "bad" bacteria entering the bloodstream and endotoxin produced from the "bad" bacteria create similar conditions because they both activate the immune system.

Endotoxin is part of the outer membrane of a type of bacteria known as the Gram-negative bacteria. Examples of Gram-negative bacteria would include *E. coli*, *Pseudomonas*, and *Klebsiella*, among others. As noted above, "endo" means "inside the body," and, of course, "toxin" means "poison," so we are literally being poisoned from the inside out. Endotoxin (LPS) is initially released from the bacterial cell wall when the cell dies or makes copies of itself. In less common scenarios, high impact exercise like marathon running can actually cause damage to the bacterial cells, leading to release of endotoxin. When undigested starch or soluble fiber reaches the large intestine, this becomes a food source for the Gram-negative bacteria, which allows them to continue to make copies of themselves and release more endotoxin.

It's important to note that the intestinal lining is only one cell thick. Being only one cell thick, it doesn't take much to damage it. The body protects the intestinal lining with a multi-layered mucosal barrier that ordinarily keeps the microbiome bacteria a safe distance away from the lining. Anything that disrupts this mucosal barrier or causes inflammation to the intestinal wall has the potential for creating serious and significant health problems.

If just a small amount of endotoxin is released—as happens in normal digestion and if the liver is working just fine—the liver will breakdown the endotoxin, and the endotoxin will be excreted out of the body without causing any significant systemic symptoms. However, if there is too much endotoxin created, the endotoxin will cause marked irritation and increased inflammation of the intestinal lining by penetrating the mucosal barrier. As we talked about earlier regarding "leaky gut syndrome," the endotoxin will then be allowed to migrate through the intestinal lining and get into the bloodstream. If a person already has an inflamed intestinal wall (like from chronic stress, excess alcohol, or food intolerance from gluten), then more and more endotoxin will be released into the bloodstream. This will, in turn, cause more intestinal wall inflammation; now we are starting to create serious problems.

As the endotoxin irritates the intestinal wall, this irritation increases both the production and the release of serotonin. Serotonin is one of the body's main neurotransmitters thought to be responsible for mediating stress, appetite, sleep, and mood. Unlike what most people might think, the vast majority of the body's serotonin is actually made in the GI tract—up to 90%, with only 10% of the body's serotonin located in the brain. For the moment, we will ignore serotonin's effects in the brain but will instead focus on the effects of serotonin on the rest of the body. Serotonin can cause symptoms such as clotting, flushing, and/or diarrhea.

Serotonin in the body increases with a chronic stress response and is one of the primary mediators of fibrosis-scarring of tissue within an organ. Studies show a strong link between serotonin and chronic conditions like diabetes, obesity, and insulin resistance.[1] Pharmaceutical companies are now running drug trials to inhibit levels of serotonin in order to attempt to treat diabetes and obesity.

Once endotoxin makes its way into the bloodstream, it acts on a specific receptor, the TLR4, which stands for *toll-like receptor 4*. This receptor is part of the immune system. Its main purpose is to recognize and signal the immune system to create an inflammatory response activating inflammatory cytokines. When endotoxin (LPS) binds to the TLR4, this also causes an allergic response through the release of histamine.[2]

Let's look at some specific health problems that endotoxin creates. Researchers have found that in otherwise healthy people, endotoxin can trigger heart attacks and/or strokes and could also play a role in Alzheimer's disease, osteoarthritis, rheumatoid arthritis, and/or diabetes. As referenced above, research shows that Gram-negative bacteria and endotoxin (LPS) are present in larger numbers in Alzheimer's disease; research also shows that endotoxin (LPS) is actually found to be present in the amyloid plaques that are responsible for the neuropathology of Alzheimer's disease.[3]

According to a Yale study published in 2016 in the journal Science, bacteria from the gut was found to trigger autoimmune conditions that could be treated and reversed with antibiotics. This makes one wonder if we can extrapolate these to other autoimmune conditions, including a long list of diseases, such as lupus, rheumatoid arthritis, psoriasis, multiple sclerosis, autoimmune liver disease, thyroid disease, and the list goes on and on.

Endotoxin also has what is described as a GELDING effect, which stands for *Gut Endotoxin Leading Decline in Gonadal function*. This seems to imply that endotoxin has an inhibitory effect on the gonads (testicles) and/or the pituitary gland to lower testosterone (circulating androgens) to low levels similar to those found in castrated men.[4] Endotoxin has also been found to have the same effect on the ovaries of women, decreasing levels of progesterone. The authors of the research study identifying the GELDING effect blamed this effect on fat. They stated that a high fat diet resulted in the gut barrier breakdown and inflammation which thereby increased endotoxin absorption into the bloodstream.[5]

So, a certain type of dietary fat can cause inflammation and can contribute to endotoxin's release into the bloodstream, but we know that there are other types of fat that are actually protective. In Parts Two and Three of this book, we will teach you which fats to avoid and which fats help in healing the body.

We know that endotoxin is one of the most detrimental GI byproducts with regard to your overall health. We will go into greater detail in the third part of this book, talking about how we can eat to eliminate and prevent the inflammation associated with endotoxin. In fact, one of the main functions of our plan is to heal the GI tract, by increasing the quality of digestion, decreasing inflammation, and reducing endotoxin.

Food probably plays the biggest role in optimal GI health and/or dysfunction. The food we consume can itself have a detrimental effect on the intestinal lining as it travels through the digestive tract. It can also feed the "bad" bacteria and thereby increase endotoxin. In the microbiome research community, everybody agrees that the gut is a key to our overall health and wellbeing, but there is not a consensus of the best way in which to achieve that healthy microbiome.

We all have heard that we should eat fiber for a healthy gut. But there are various types of fiber. Is all fiber equally important, or is there a particular type of fiber that is most beneficial to our digestive tract? Let's look more at what fiber actually is. Fiber is another type of carbohydrate that cannot be digested by human digestive enzymes.[6] As a result, it makes its way through the digestive tract to the large intestine intact. There are two classifications of fiber—soluble fiber and insoluble fiber. Soluble fiber can be digested by all bacteria in the large intestine through the process of fermentation—exactly how we make beer and wine. In the case of soluble fiber fermentation, the process creates short-chain fatty acids that can be absorbed into the bloodstream and used as fuel. As this fermentation happens, it is feeding the bacteria, both the "good" and "bad" bacteria, at the same time. Feeding the "bad" bacteria produces endotoxin, which may not be detrimental to a person with a healthy intestinal lining, but it can be disastrous to a person with a compromised intestinal lining or other form of intestinal inflammation.

Insoluble fiber is not digestible by any of the bacteria in the large intestine. It works more like a broom to sweep out the bad bacteria. This is the type of fiber that we want to eat a lot of. In fact, hunter-gatherer peoples throughout thousands of years of history have eaten root vegetables, most of which have a naturally high content of insoluble fiber. Because our ancestors did not have grains readily available, which make up most of our fiber today, insoluble fiber was a large source of their food supply. We're going to talk more later about how we can use fiber in our diet to create a healthier microbiome.

Speaking of grains, we mentioned gluten earlier and how some people are allergic and/or intolerant to it. Gluten is actually a *lectin*, which is a protein found in wheat, rye, barley, and some oats. Lectins are a type of protein that can bind to *polysaccharides* (carbohydrates). Gluten is indigestible by humans. Even if a person was not intolerant to gluten, gluten still irritates the intestinal lining and creates inflammation. As if that were not bad enough, most of the grains that we eat have been sprayed with pesticides, including one that is a well-known carcinogen, Roundup (glyphosate). Roundup is so toxic that Europe has banned its use and will not accept our grain products for use in their food supply; we, however, still use it on crops here that are not organically grown. We will go into greater detail about lectins and how to avoid the different types of lectin/gluten in our diet/nutrition section.

In spite of all we hear about gluten and its toxic effects on the GI tract, perhaps the most detrimental food that affects the intestinal lining is a certain type of fat, PUFA (short for polyunsaturated fatty acid). We will talk extensively about PUFA in the diet/nutrition section of our plan. This does not mean that all fats are bad. In fact, there are certain types of fat that are greatly beneficial to our overall health and to the GI tract. An example is the avocado, which is a type of monounsaturated fatty acid. Coconut oil is another example of a healthy fat; it is a saturated fatty acid. We will be discussing healthy fats as a major part of an optimal diet in the diet/nutrition section of this book, but as there is much debate and controversy, the discussion around PUFA and healthy fats will take up their own chapter.

Undigested protein also feeds the bacteria, which is why the health of the gut starts in the stomach with healthy hydrochloric acid production to break down protein. We will cover how to increase stomach acid later on in our plan for healthy digestion. If undigested protein makes it down to the large intestine, then there will likely be an increase in inflammatory processes within the digestive tract.

Emulsifiers in food are another contributor to gut lining irritation. These are not normally ingested substances, although they may be naturally occurring. Ingredients such as various gums acting mainly as thickeners in the food product are perhaps the most well-known emulsifiers. The most commonly used emulsifier is *carrageenan*. There are many others. One or more of these compounds can be found in most commercially processed foods, including the "healthy organic foods." Studies show that even in low concentrations, these substances damage the mucosa of the large intestine, creating lesions that lead to the inflammatory openings we discussed earlier.

This inflammation allows for both endotoxin and bacteria to enter the bloodstream and to translocate to the brain. As a result of the inflammation from ingestion of these emulsifiers, researchers have found that when endotoxin activates the inflammatory TLR4 pathway, this causes a certain type of brain tumor known as *cerebral cavernoma* or *cerebral cavernous malformation* (CVM).[7] This type of tumor can cause seizures and hemorrhagic strokes. It has also been shown in mouse studies that low amounts of emulsifiers produce low-grade inflammation, obesity, and even metabolic syndrome.[8]

As mentioned earlier, carbohydrates also feed the bacteria in the gut. This is where there is much confusion. It is true that if starch makes it to the large intestine, it will feed the bacteria and create more endotoxin. But there is a caveat to this. Most carbohydrates are digested and absorbed in the small intestine, so only the undigested carbohydrates presenting in the large intestine will cause a problem. Many people will say that you should eat "complex" carbohydrates and not eat "simple" carbohydrates, such as sugar and/or fruit, because they break down quickly and are rapidly absorbed. But in the case of a person with a gastrointestinal problem or "bad" bacteria overgrowth, simple carbohydrates are a good thing because these types of carbohydrates will never reach the large intestine undigested to feed the bacteria. The more complex carbohydrates, such as whole grains, though they may have more nutrients, may not be fully digested in the small intestine, and, therefore, undigested portions may reach the large intestine and produce more endotoxin and, as a result, more inflammation. We will be talking more about the different types of carbohydrates in Part Two of this book.

There is also a class of starch found in some foods known as resistant starch. This is a starch that the body is unable to digest in the small intestine and needs the bacteria present in the large intestine to digest. There are some good qualities about this particular type of starch. It is known to lower cholesterol, and, when it is fermented by the bacteria in the large intestine, it produces a chemical known as *butyrate*, which is a short-chain fatty acid that the body can actually use for fuel.

When we speak of ketogenic (low carb) diets, one of the main benefits that people report is feeling much better at the beginning of the diet. They will report having less bloating, less swelling, and significant weight loss. They may also feel less fatigued, have fewer headaches, and have fewer sugar and carb cravings. This is mainly because, when they eliminate carbohydrates from their diet, they have invariably reduced the soluble fiber and resistant starch that make their way to the large intestine to feed the Gram-negative bacteria. This in itself is telling in diagnosing what is happening with the microbiome.

So, as with any type of food, this is where we have to decide on an individual basis if it's better to have a more nutritious food that can increase endotoxin or a less nutritious food that will not. This will be an important discussion and a significant part of the theme found in the second half of this book. The microbiome is so diverse from one person to another that any food that is healthy to one may be a poison to another. This is why, people who say that one type of diet is good for everyone have not accounted for all the possibilities that may be different for each individual. As we move forward, we will help you to know which foods may be good for you. Even when all the experts say you just need to eat less to lose weight, they are not considering the most updated research showing how much the gut microbiome and inflammation matter when it comes to weight loss and/or weight gain.

## Takeaways from Chapter 9

1. Endotoxin (*lipopolysaccharide*) is a toxin released by "bad" bacteria in the large intestine and can be an underlying factor in many autoimmune disorders.

2. If there is too much endotoxin created, the endotoxin will cause marked irritation and increased inflammation of the intestinal lining by penetrating the mucosal barrier.

3. Food is the biggest contributor for optimal GI health and/or dysfunction. The food we consume can contribute to the growth of "bad" bacteria and thereby an increase in endotoxin.

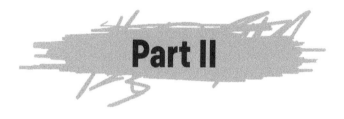

# Part II

## Diets and Dieting

Diagramming

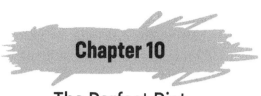

# Chapter 10

## The Perfect Diet

Now that you know about all the problems that too much stress can cause (i.e., increasing the stress/aging hormones cortisol, estrogen, and insulin) we can begin to talk about how to interrupt the cycle. We've also discussed the catastrophic negative effects that GI tract dysfunction can have and the role it and inflammation play in poor health. The good news is that we can stop all these negative effects dead in their tracks. And, even better, we can reverse the damage that has already been done.

Our first focus of the plan will be diet. Why? Because diet and nutrition have the greatest effect on every aspect of our body and our health. We all have to eat, so what we take in every day is the biggest life changer. What we eat is either making us healthier or making us sicker. What we eat affects our mood, our ability to think, whether we have energy for the day, or whether we are worn out before we get started. If we are eating a poor diet, it will cause serious problems, such as heart disease, diabetes, autoimmune conditions, and, yes, even cancer. Of course, what we choose to eat every day can also determine whether we are skinny or whether we are fat.

Another important clarification—in this book when we use the word "diet," we are using it in the context of what we eat, not in the same way that it is often used to refer to dieting or weight loss. The way of eating that we are discussing here is not a "lose weight" diet specifically; rather, it is a "get healthy" diet because we know that the weight will come off naturally as the body returns to a state of more optimal health.

How much we eat is important, as we talked about earlier. Eating more calories than your metabolism can support will interfere with weight loss; however, not eating enough calories will slow your metabolism, increase your stress response, and pack on the pounds. So, how do we determine how many calories we need to eat? In part, it will be based on your metabolism. The first thing we need to do is avoid any type of diet focused on fasting, even intermittent fasting—at least at the beginning. We are trying to avoid inflammation and triggering the body's stress response. A good guideline for daily caloric intake would be around 2,200 calories for men and 1,800 calories for women; this could be more, but this is a fair starting point.

One of the critical ideas we want to highlight with this book is that we become overweight by becoming unhealthy, so the key is to get healthy in order to lose the weight, not lose the weight in order to get healthy.

This idea is a mistake that many people make. If we can learn to think of being overweight as a *symptom* rather than a problem, then we will take the correct action(s) in order to get our desired results. What we eat should be actively helping us decrease systemic inflammation, definitely not increasing inflammation.

The diet should be anti-stress, to keep us from going into a "fight or flight" stress response. When we eat too few calories for our metabolism, we start releasing cortisol; having too few calories becomes a signal to the body that we are starving, and the body will, therefore, begin to conserve energy and store fat.

A healthy diet should support balanced hormones, which we will get when we eat foods that will limit the stress response, maximize the anti-aging hormones, and minimize the aging hormones. Also, avoiding PUFA will go a long way in balancing out the hormones.

Another important benefit of a healthy diet is its ability to maintain a healthy gut and not feed the "bad" bacteria in the colon that produce endotoxin, which poisons us. This detrimental process often leads to the development of autoimmune conditions, like rheumatoid arthritis, Hashimoto's thyroiditis, lupus, Crohn's disease, and/or ulcerative colitis.

The diet should be maintainable—if you can only stick to the diet plan for a short time, then it will obviously not be a long-term solution. We are going for changes that we can sustain over a longer term. The goal of any healthy diet is the long-term benefits, as opposed to a quick fix or losing enough weight just to get into that dress or suit for the high school reunion or wedding that is coming up in a few weeks.

Therefore, the perfect diet for us would be an all-natural, unprocessed diet. If we look at the history and research of native peoples from around the world who ate or continue to eat their natural diets, we find that they are healthy—with little to no obesity, no heart disease, no diabetes, and no autoimmune conditions. One researcher from the 1930s, Dr. Weston Price, was a dentist who wanted to discover the causes for the change in dental health in modern cultures. He looked at cultures who had switched from a traditional diet to a "modern" diet. He compiled his research in a 528-page book titled *Nutrition and Physical Degeneration*. Dr. Price traveled around the world looking at various cultures and saw that within one generation of adopting a "modern" diet, the people had gone from having minimal dental cavities, perfect dental arches, and overall excellent health to having deformed jaws, multiple cavities, crooked teeth, and overall poor health. The main reason for the change in health, according to Dr. Price, was the change in diet from unprocessed to processed foods.

We think it is only common sense, and we believe most people will agree, that eating unprocessed, whole foods is a healthier way to eat—although, in our fast-paced, stressful society, eating healthy is much easier said than done. With packaged food, we see ingredients that resemble a science project, getting further and further away from the more natural, unprocessed foods that our ancestors ate. Add in all the chemicals that are sprayed on the crops, and the chemicals that are involved in packaging the food, and now we have food that is basically devoid of nutrients and full of empty calories. This is what is meant when we hear the leading experts in nutrition tell us that as Americans, we are a "nation of overfed and undernourished people."[1]

One type of diet that has become popular as of late is called a "paleo," or primal, diet. The premise is to eat like a caveman/cavewoman, avoiding all foods of "modern" humans. Paleo gurus advise us to eliminate all dairy, all grains, all starchy vegetables such as potatoes, and eliminate most fruits because Paleolithic humans did not have these to eat. Foods these diets recommend are meats, nuts, and vegetables—low carbs. In general, the theory behind eating this way makes a good starting point for dietary modifications. However, one of the knocks against a paleo diet is that many of the proponents and many of the book authors are dogmatic and recommend eliminating many foods that can be beneficial, even though they are "modern" foods. A paleo or primal diet eliminates some healthy foods, like many fruits and vegetables, that may not have been present in primitive times but are still nutrient-rich. Such a diet, in general, is the basis for a clean diet but tends to be so restrictive that people have trouble following it; furthermore, it becomes difficult to stick with it for the long term. When people are strictly following the paleo diet, they often turn their daily intake into a low-calorie, low-carb diet that can altogether cause problems.

Another problem with a paleo diet is that we are not totally sure what Paleolithic people ate, and we may not even have access to the same types of food they ate. It could mean they were missing some key nutrients. Also, as we mentioned above, it is often difficult to get enough daily calories with a paleo diet, since it tends to be low carb. The theory that primitive humans ate low carb may also be false, since some researchers show that root vegetables (sweet potatoes, yams, brown potatoes) may have been a main dietary component for Ice Age humans. Many people think one group of people in particular, the Innuits, living in what is now modern-day Alaska, do not consume any carbs, but they are able to consume glucose in the form of glycogen, which is present in the fresh meat and fish they eat raw or frozen. We are not able to do this when we eat store-bought meat, because of the enzymes that degrade the glycogen as it's aging. If modern humans want to eat like the Paleolithic peoples, then we would eat all parts of the animal. Traditional cultures would eat from nose to tail. We see this in different cultures even today.

We're not suggesting that we eat this way. However, one important benefit of eating all parts of the animal is consuming the collagen and bone marrow. Most Americans only eat muscle meat. We do not usually eat organ meat such as liver, kidney, gizzards, tongue, testicles, heart, and brains. Organ meat is where many of the nutrients are, especially the fat-soluble vitamins. Since we typically eat only muscle meat, we are missing out on many of these key vitamins. Only recently has bone broth become popular. Bone broth is made by cooking bones for many hours so as to release the bone marrow to make it into a broth. This is a great source of nutrients, and many cultures still make this with dishes such as ox tail soup, chicken feet soup, and good old chicken soup made with the whole chicken.

For many people, eating a strict diet of just meat and vegetables becomes socially restrictive and boring. As we go through the plan, we will also stress eating a variety of unprocessed, whole foods, making it practical to follow in our modern world without any feeling of deprivation.

## Benefits of a Healthy Diet

What are the benefits of a healthy diet? It all depends on the lens we look through. The geneticist will look at how it affects our genes, and a longevity doctor will look at how it increases the length of our telomeres. (Telomeres are those little end caps on the ends of DNA strands that are needed for producing more cells.) In addition, there are certain popular diets focusing mainly on weight loss that will decrease testosterone and progesterone and increase cortisol and estrogen. In many cases, a person will follow a diet for two weeks until they lose ten pounds and then they gain it all back when they return to eating "normally," and, at that point, it's time to start another "latest and greatest diet."

The lens that we want you to look through is the bioenergetic model, which means that what we are eating should provide us with all the energy that our body needs to grow, repair, and function at its best. As a result of a healthy diet and lifestyle, our brain will have all the energy it needs to solve complex problems, to be creative, and to feel happy and alert. If you have ever had low blood sugar, you may have had symptoms of becoming lightheaded ("brain fog" or "spacey") because the brain uses a lot of energy. So, we want to have enough energy for a highly functioning brain.

But before we start talking about what we need to do to optimize our diet, we first need to debunk some common myths and define some basic concepts (so we are all on the same page when we start discussing how to eat). This may seem like basic information for some, but, with all the misinformation and disinformation available these days, it is better not to assume.

## Debunking Some Common Myths

- There is not one diet that is perfect for everyone, but there are some truths that are true for everyone. We can all probably agree that exposure to radiation is not good, and we all know the dangers of smoking. This is the same for certain foods that we must learn to avoid, those that are toxic to us.

- One of the most common questions people ask is, "Can you just give me a food plan and let me follow it? I don't need all the science." After working with thousands of people, we know that if a person does not understand the reasoning behind the recommendation, the plan may not make any sense and there will likely not be any consistent follow-through. When they hear about the latest and greatest "new diet" that their hairdresser tells them about, they will forget about the food plan they're supposed to be following. Or if they have not lost twenty pounds in the first two weeks, they will quickly say this is "not working" for them. This is exactly why the weight loss/dieting market makes billions of dollars—because it is not necessarily based on science or facts; it's tailored to people's emotions, and people rarely get the lasting results they are promised.

- Most people who are overweight say they have lost and gained hundreds of pounds over the decades in their never-ending, yo-yo dieting. They lose twenty pounds, rave about the diet they're on, only to regain it all back and then some when they return to "normal" eating. They repeat this behavior over and over with the latest and greatest "diet" in a never-ending cycle. This cycle causes them to feel like a failure because they either could not stick to the plan or because the plan did not work for them. If we think about weight loss in a logical way, we should remember that it took us years to put on a certain amount of fat and a certain amount of weight, so how or why would it all come off in just a few weeks?

- A general rule of thumb—fat lost slowly is more likely to be permanent fat loss, whereas fat lost quickly is destined to return, plus more.

- We will discuss how it is not all about "calories in versus calories out" like the diet gurus and mainstream media would have you believe, but it is more about foods that cause inflammation, that inhibit our thyroid hormones, that inhibit our metabolism, and that increase the "bad" intestinal bacteria.

Once we eliminate stress and inflammation by following the plan we are outlining in this book, once we provide the body with proper nutrients and energy to balance out the hormones, and once we work to remove the inflammatory foods from our diet, the body will most likely shed the fat naturally without us having to starve ourselves.

---

## Takeaways from Chapter 10

1. Americans are a "nation of overfed and undernourished people." What we are eating should provide us with all the energy that our body needs to grow, repair, and function at its best.

2. Bone broth is a great source of collagen and many other nutrients essential to optimal health and wellness.

3. Focusing our diet on unprocessed, whole foods is essential for good health and optimal energy. There is not one specific diet that is perfect for everyone.

---

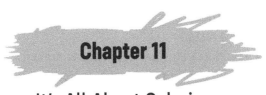

# Chapter 11

# It's All About Calories

## Eat Enough to Lose Weight; Starve to Gain Weight

Let's look at why getting enough calories every day can be such a big game changer for people who chronically diet.

Some scientists have performed experiments with earthworms, finding that if the earthworms eat a minimal, near starvation-level diet, this increases their life span.[1] Not sure about you, but who wants to live longer if you're feeling lethargic and hungry all the time, and if your hormones are unbalanced, making you depressed, moody, and anxious?

Remember that the main energy and main metabolism hormone is the thyroid hormone. We talked about this in Chapter 6. If you have an abundance of active thyroid hormone (T3), and if your body is able to utilize the hormone as intended, then you will have a faster metabolism, and you'll have more energy than someone with low thyroid function. A faster metabolism means you burn more calories at rest. We all know that person with a fast metabolism who everyone hates, who can eat whatever they want and not gain an ounce. We see this most often in children and teenagers.

However, when a person is dieting, either acutely or chronically, it decreases the amount of active thyroid hormone circulating within the body by up to 50%, which, in turn, reduces the resting metabolism rate by anywhere from 15 to 40%! Just to maintain your current weight with this type of decrease, you would need to cut 40% of your calories. This can mean the difference between eating a diet of 2,400 calories per day versus 1,440 calories per day, which is an adaptive process the body uses to conserve energy. Unfortunately, the decrease in our metabolism when we diet lasts long after the dieting is over! People who chronically diet may never have their thyroid hormone levels return to normal. And so often, this decrease in our thyroid hormones from chronically dieting will not be picked up through normal laboratory tests.

If we tell you that you may need to eat more calories in order to lose the weight you are trying to lose, we know that you won't believe us! We know you've heard from nearly every source that if you are going to lose weight, you have to dramatically lower your calorie intake, but this is just not the case. If you really want to lose the weight without putting it all back on later, plus some, you will need to take in an adequate number of calories every day that will enable your body to increase its resting metabolic rate. Studies show that 95% of people dieting through prolonged calorie deprivation will fail to achieve lasting results. Stephen Guyenet, PhD, who is a neurobiologist and obesity researcher, stated the following:

> If there's one thing that's consistent in the medical literature, it's that telling people to eat fewer calories does not help them lose weight in the long term. Many people who use this strategy see transient fat loss, followed by fat regain and a feeling of defeat. There's a simple reason for it: the body doesn't want to lose weight. It's extremely difficult to fight the fat mass set-point, and the body will use every tool it has to maintain its preferred level of fat: hunger, reduced body temperature, higher muscle efficiency (i.e., less energy is expended for the same movement), lethargy, lowered immune function, et cetera.[2]

To prove this point, you don't typically see a reunion show for a show like *The Biggest Loser*. If you are not familiar with the show, it's a reality television show that's based on a competition between grossly overweight men and women in a bootcamp type of environment utilizing extreme exercise and extreme dieting. The winner is the person who loses the largest percentage of their body weight. People who compete usually lose extreme amounts of weight in a relatively short period of time. The problem is when these people leave the show and stop the extreme dieting and exercise, they gain all of the weight back, plus some.

Just illustrating what we are talking about, the contestants have been using the extreme exercise to artificially raise their metabolism, which is inherently slow. The extreme exercise does nothing to reset their metabolism long term. In fact, once they stop the exercise, and it's no longer there to burn the calories, their metabolism slows to its original set point, and all the weight comes back. Reports show that 90% of *The Biggest Loser* participants regain all the weight they initially lost.

It's really not a surprise at all. We know that this type of extreme dieting and exercise slows an already slow metabolism, and we know that any type of artificial increase in the metabolism is not sustainable over time. We see this in professional athletes. Often, when an athlete retires from their sport, soon afterward, they gain tremendous amounts of weight and often develop many health conditions. You probably know these types of people, who, if they are not running their five to ten miles several times per week, are gaining weight. It means they can never stop; it is like being on a treadmill where you must always keep walking to stay in one place.

So, the goal is not to slow our already slowed metabolism, but to increase our resting metabolism through taking in enough calories while we are balancing out the hormones—i.e., increasing the anti-aging hormones, decreasing the aging hormones, and addressing any or all issues that contribute to any decreases in our metabolism. Although it's common for our metabolism to decrease as we age, this is not necessarily natural, and the body will reset to a higher metabolism with time.

## Reasons Why Not to Diet:
### The Minnesota Starvation Experiment (1945)

One of the best research studies to show the longer-term effects of chronic dieting is The Minnesota Starvation Experiment. This study was published at the end of World War II in 1945. It was conducted to study the effects of starvation and was attempting to mimic the effects that starvation was having on the European population as a result of decreased availability of food during the war. However, this was a one-of-a-kind study on humans, because once the significant negative side effects began to show up—severe depression, anxiety, and mental instability—it would be deemed unethical by today's research standards. The study recruited a group of thirty-six young men who were conscientious war objectors. They could opt to be part of this experiment instead of going to war.

The study was broken up into four parts:

1. The Control Phase: For twelve weeks, the men were fed a 3,200-calorie diet each day. At the end of this phase, they were deemed slightly under weight.

2. Semi-Starvation Phase: For the following twenty-four weeks, each person's dietary intake was reduced to 1,560 calories per day. Think about this in terms of today's caloric intake and how most people who are trying to lose weight are eating under 1,000–1,200 calories per day.

3. Restricted Rehab Phase: For an additional twelve weeks, they were divided into four groups with different calorie intakes, ranging from 2,000 to 3,200 calories per day.

4. Unrestriced Rehab Phase: In the last eight weeks of the experiment, they were allowed to eat whatever they wanted, and calories were unrestricted.

All study subjects were also exercising daily—they walked twenty-two miles per week. Results were published in a two-volume, 1,385-page report, *The Biology of Human Starvation*. The conclusions that this semi-starvation experiment produced include the following:

- periods of extreme emotional distress and depression
- increases in hysteria and hypochondria
- a preoccupation with food during both the starvation and rehab phases
- drastically decreased sex drive
- anxiety, along with social withdrawal
- decrease in focus, decreased concentration, and difficulties with comprehension (even though on standardized tests, there was no indication of any mental decline)[3]

These results seem to indicate that participants' deficits were mainly perceived and subjective, versus actual and observed. There were, however, observable changes in their physiology, such as a decreased metabolic rate, evidenced by decreased body temperature, decreased respiration, and decreased heart rate. Some of the volunteers showed signs of edema in their extremities. Most all of the volunteers became obsessed with eating, and, during the refeeding phase, many ate continuously.

When the volunteers were refeeding, they all gained weight, exceeding where they started the experiment, and then, after time within months, they settled back to their normal, pre-experiment weight. This was seen as part of the healing process.

It's interesting that these are many of the same symptoms we see in people that are dieting to lose weight. Some dieters start to feel better almost immediately once they start eating more calories. Remember, the Minnesota study subjects' normal caloric intake was 3,200 calories per day, and their "starvation" intake was 1,560 calories per day. This is more calories per day than most people who diet today eat. In fact, you can see weight loss programs featured on TV that recommend diets as low as 1,200 calories per day.

Though we know that cortisol, hormones, and inflammation are the main controllers for weight gain and will impact our ability to regulate our weight, we still cannot forget about calories entirely. This being said, we don't want to focus only on calories, but, since many people do, let's look at how misguided this can be, especially when people are looking for a quick way to lose fat. Many people tell us that they lost twenty pounds in two weeks on some type of diet, only to gain the twenty pounds back plus another ten pounds in the process. We know automatically that their weight loss was predominantly water and/or muscle, but it was not fat loss.

Let's do a little math and use logic. One pound of fat is equivalent to approximately 3,500 calories. This means to lose one pound of fat, you would need to burn 3,500 calories more than you consume over any period of time. That would mean to lose one pound per week (without accounting for any slowed metabolism or other metabolic influences), you would need to drop your daily caloric intake by 500 calories a day (500 calories x 7 days = 3,500 calories). Basically, you would be taking in 1,500 calories per day if normally eating a 2,000-calorie-per-day diet. This is fairly doable and relatively sustainable over time.

However, many people who chronically diet have actually lowered their basal metabolic rate (in layman's terms, their "resting metabolic rate"). This rate determines how many calories a day we burn for fuel. Slowing of the resting metabolic rate happens as a result of the chronic dieting, which, in turn, contributes to a chronic stress response. A chronic stress response creates higher cortisol levels. This rise in cortisol levels increases the storage of central body fat, while also increasing the burning of muscle, neither of which is the desired outcome, and both of which, ironically, contribute to more weight gain. A lot of people are currently following various dietary recommendations of 1,200 calories per day in an attempt to facilitate weight loss. But, as we are seeing, what actually tends to happen is people gain more weight, not lose it. We see that with a slower resting metabolic rate of around 1,200 calories per day, it is physically impossible to sustain a two-pound-per-week weight loss over time. In order to sustain this kind of weight loss over time, it would require that a person eat nothing at all, which would further decrease their resting metabolic rate.

A better goal and more sustainable weight loss over time would be a target of one-half to one pound per week. However, the emotional drive to lose fat is so strong that people tend to focus mainly on the amount of weight lost and not the sustainability. It is well known by researchers that those who are losing weight quickly are doing so at the expense of their muscle mass, creating a significant stress response, and, therefore, the weight lost is generally mostly water weight and muscle mass, not the desired fat loss.

## You Have to Eat to Increase Your Metabolism

Another factor with chronic dieters is that when they start healing, restoring, and increasing their metabolic rate, they will initially gain weight and go above where they started until their metabolism is restored. It's only at that point that they will start losing weight. This result has been demonstrated in many studies, which makes sense if you think about it.

If you have slowed your metabolism down to around 1,200 calories per day, and you need to eat more calories to improve your metabolism—say 2,000 calories—of course your metabolism will not change overnight. The extra calories will initially be stored as fat. This is just a part of the healing process.

An analogy can be made to a person who starts exercising and is sore for a few days later. This is just part of the adaptive mechanism and does not in any way mean that exercise is bad for you because it made you sore. We always have to remind ourselves that this is the way the body works. Many people become discouraged as soon as they gain a pound. They automatically want to decrease the calories in order to lose the weight, and there they go—right back on the weight loss merry-go-round. Unfortunately, this is how the idea of dieting is working in our society right now. We all know that you can't sell a diet plan by telling people they will gain weight.

The main point is you must eat to increase your metabolism and to minimize any stress response, in order to preserve and build muscle while losing fat and decreasing inflammation.

---

## Takeaways from Chapter 11

1. In order to raise our metabolism, we must ensure we eat enough and are getting adequate calories every day.

2. Extreme dieting and extreme exercising actually slows our metabolism, making it easier to gain weight and harder to lose weight.

3. You have to eat more, not fewer, calories if you want to lose weight!

# Chapter 12

## Food Groups

### So, What Should We Eat?

We will start by going over a few basics. Food nutrients can be classified by their macro-nutrients and by their micronutrients. "Macro" means "large," and these nutrients are divided into three groups—protein, carbohydrates, and fat. "Micro" means "small," so this would be the smaller nutrients like vitamins, minerals, and trace minerals. We often talk about the micronutrients as supplements, and we will be discussing those later in the book.

Let's start with the macronutrients. Most everyone has heard of protein, carbs, and fats, but let's go ahead and define them, as they will be the mainstay of our daily diet/food plan.

### Protein

Protein is an essential nutrient, meaning we cannot live without it. Proteins are the building blocks of the body. They are used to build muscle and make and repair tissue. In addition, they are the source of all the enzymes involved in the many metabolic processes throughout the body. As you learned earlier in the book, protein can also be converted into energy when the body is under stress or when the body is low in carbohydrates. Proteins are made up of individual amino acids that are attached in long chains. When protein is digested, it is eventually broken down into these individual amino acids.

There are twenty different amino acids, nine of which are essential, meaning that you must get them from your diet. They are histidine, leucine, phenylalanine, lysine, theanine, isoleucine, methionine, valine, and tryptophan. The other eleven non-essential amino acids can actually be made by converting one amino acid into another. Protein is found most abundantly in animal products such as meat, dairy, and eggs. It can also be found in some vegetables. If a food contains all the essential amino acids, it is considered a "complete protein." The proteins from animal products contain all the essential amino acids. Plants, for the most part, are missing one or more of the essential amino acids, so they are mostly considered "incomplete proteins." There is some debate whether certain grains such as quinoa are considered complete or incomplete proteins. Therefore, if a person is a vegetarian, they must combine different plant foods in order to get a mixture of all the essential amino acids.

Currently, there is not a consensus of how much protein a person needs per day. Some experts will say, on average, 0.8 grams per kilogram of body weight or as high as 2 grams per kilogram for athletes. Most people need at least 1.2 g/kg of their body weight. For a person weighing 150 pounds, this would be roughly 82 g of protein per day. Signs of protein deficiency are diarrhea, failure to thrive, inability to heal injuries, fatty liver, and swelling in the abdomen, legs, and feet.

## Carbohydrates

As mentioned earlier in Part One, carbohydrates are the primary energy source for the body. Carbs are sugars, starches, and fibers found in fruits and vegetables. Even though they have garnered a bad reputation lately by many in the mainstream media and by the "low-carb" proponents, carbohydrates are not only the primary energy source for the body—but they are the preferred energy source. If the body has carbs, it will preferentially use them for fuel first.

Carbs are converted into ATP, the body's main form of energy, in a complicated three-step process. The three steps are glycolysis, the Krebs cycle, and the electron transport chain. The end results are ATP, carbon dioxide ($CO_2$), and water. All three byproducts are especially important to your health. Of course, we all know the importance of energy and water, but carbon dioxide is also essential. Many people in the healthcare field consider carbon dioxide to be a waste product.

Carbohydrates produce the most carbon dioxide, followed by proteins, followed by fats, which produce the least $CO_2$. When there is less $CO_2$ around, this will increase the production of lactic acid, promoting inflammation and fibrosis. Although it seems contrary to what we might expect, high $CO_2$ levels actually increase the amount of oxygen that can readily enter any of the cells in the body. It's important to note that $CO_2$ is needed for oxygen to be available to the cells.

Carbs are commonly divided into two groups: "simple carbs" and "complex carbs." We talked briefly about these in Chapter 9. Simple carbs are the smaller molecules, the *monosaccharides* ("mono" means "one," and "saccharide" means "sugar," so, "single sugars") and the *disaccharides* ("di" means "two," so, "two sugars"). The monosaccharides are glucose, fructose, and galactose. Then we have the disaccharides, which are made up of two molecules: *sucrose*, which is sugar (glucose and fructose) and *lactose* (galactose and glucose), i.e., "milk sugar." Included in the simple carbohydrates are the sugars found in all alcoholic drinks. The complex carbs are larger molecules, which include starches and fibers. We also talked about the benefits of starches and fibers in Chapters 8 and 9. Starches are basically composed of long strands of glucose molecules. Starches and fibers are found in beans, potatoes, other vegetables, fruits, and whole grains.

All carbohydrates eventually break down to the single molecule sugars of glucose, fructose, and/or galactose. It does not matter whether you eat a piece of whole wheat toast or a candy bar; both will break down to a single molecule of glucose. What is different is the speed at which they break down to these single molecules. The complex carbs break down more slowly than the simple carbs, which provides a steadier stream of glucose for energy production. Once the carbs are broken down to glucose, they can then be used and converted into the body's main energy source, ATP.

Every cell in the body can use glucose for energy. Some cells can use only glucose, such as nerve tissue and red blood cells. As we talked about earlier, glucose is so important to the body that when there is not enough glucose in the bloodstream, the body will convert protein into glucose through a chemical process called gluconeogenesis, which we discussed earlier in Chapter 5. This is what the "low carb" proponents forget about. If the body did not prefer carbohydrates as its primary energy source, it would not have the systems in place to make the glucose in time of need.

When there is a lack of carbohydrates in the diet, the body will typically use fat as fuel to make ATP and also produce energy from byproducts of fat oxidation, namely, ketone bodies. However, don't forget that for most cells in the body, the preferential source of energy will always be carbohydrates.

## Fats

Fats and oils are technically called lipids. The term *lipid* is commonly used to refer to both the *triglycerides* and their carrier proteins, *high-density lipoprotein* (HDL), *low-density lipoprotein* (LDL), and *very-low-density lipoprotein* (VLDL). Most doctors will check your fasting lipid panel once or twice a year as a general screening for good health. Triglycerides are made up of three fatty acids connected to a glycerol molecule. Earlier, we made a point of noting that the body's preferred energy source is carbohydrates; however, fats are the main source of energy used by the muscles and the heart at rest, or during low-intensity exercise. Once the exercise reaches higher intensity, the muscles and the heart switch to burning glucose.

In addition, fats are needed for the absorption of the fat-soluble vitamins such as vitamins A, E, D, and K. Without fat, you would not be able to utilize these vitamins. Another important function of fat is to make the lipid membrane (cell wall) for just about every cell in the body. So, fat is an important component for health.

All fats are either "saturated" or "unsaturated." "Saturated fats" are made up of chains of carbon atoms without any double bonds, so they are more stable. "Unsaturated fats" are chains of carbon atoms with one or more double bonds—they are more unstable. This sounds technical, so let's talk about it in more practical terms: you can tell if a fat is saturated or unsaturated by whether it will remain solid at room temperature. If it remains solid at room temperature, then it is a saturated fat. If it turns to liquid at room temperature, then it is an unsaturated fat. (There are some exceptions.)

For our purposes in this book, we will divide fat into three different groups:

- SFA: *saturated fatty acids*
- MUFA: *mono-unsaturated fatty acids*
- PUFA: *polyunsaturated fatty acids*

As we have already talked about, SFA means there are no double bonds; MUFA, monounsaturated fat ("mono" means "one"), has one double bond; and PUFA has more than one double bond ("poly" means "more than one"). We talked a little about PUFA in Chapter 9. This will all make more sense when we begin to talk about which fats we want to eat and which fats we need to avoid.

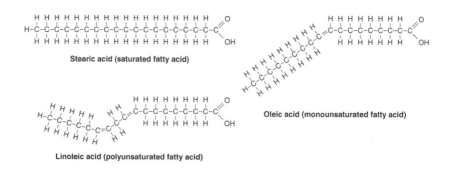

Figure 12.1. Saturated fatty acids are made up of a chain of carbon atoms without any double bonds, making them more stable. Unsaturated fats are chains of carbon atoms with one or more double bonds, making them unstable. Monounsaturated fatty acids have one double bond, while polyunsaturated fatty acids have multiple double bonds.

## Number One Health and Weight Loss Enemy—Not Sugar, but PUFA

This is not to say that all fats are bad. In fact, SFA, saturated fatty acids, and MUFA, monounsaturated fatty acids, are healthy for us. We will talk about this in the next section, where we will incorporate them into the plan. But first, let's look at how PUFA came to be such a controversial part of our diet.

## Takeaways from Chapter 12

1. The three main food groups for every meal are proteins, carbohydrates, fats.

2. Carbs are not *only* the primary energy source for the body, but they are the *preferred* energy source for the body.

3. Fats are the main source of energy used by the muscles and the heart at rest or during low intensity exercise.

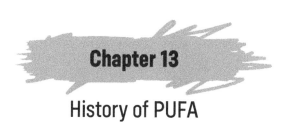

# Chapter 13

# History of PUFA

You may be asking what the big deal with PUFA is. Or you may have heard from the mainstream media that it is heart healthy, but nothing could be further from the truth.

Remember from our discussion in the fats section, Chapter 12, that PUFA stands for *polyunsaturated fatty acids*, fats that are made up of multiple double bonds and are highly unstable at room temperature. PUFA is predominantly found in all the seed and vegetable oils. This includes corn, canola, safflower, sesame, nut oils, and more. These seed and vegetable oils are referred to as omega-6 fats. Another well-known PUFA is the "heart healthy" fish oil, which is an omega-3 fat. What we are about to show will sound contradictory to what has been the mantra of the medical community and mainstream media for the past twenty years.

Now, let's take a look at the history of PUFA and how it became such a big part of our standard American diet (ironically, the "SAD" diet, no pun intended).

In the early to mid-1900s, farmers were looking for ways to fatten their livestock with cheap feed additives known as toxins. They tried using these toxins to suppress the pigs' thyroid function in order to fatten them, until they realized that the toxins were carcinogenic. Then, they tried mixing coconut oil in with the feed, but this increased the feed consumption without causing the increased weight gain that was desired. We now understand that coconut oil is thermogenic, meaning it increases metabolism, so it actually had the opposite effect. Then the farmers tried adding corn oil and soybean oil to the feed. This was a hit: it did the same as the cheap feed additives in suppressing thyroid function and allowed for rapid weight gain in the animals. Now, we are seeing that these additives are causing many health problems in people, similar to the problems they were causing in the animals.

However, the farmers were not as interested in the long-term health of the animals since they were raising them for slaughter. So, to them, these additives were a great success.

At around the same time, the Industrial Age was taking off and petroleum products were quickly replacing the seed oils in products such as paint thinners and varnishes. This was producing a glut of seed oils, and manufacturers were looking for new ways to market their products. That made the seed oils the perfect solution for farmers trying to maximize their livestock profits. With powerful seed oil lobbying and industrial use of these products no longer profitable, that brings us to where we are today.

Let's look at how different our diet and our health has become in the last 100 to 150 years since the introduction of edible seed oils to our diet—how different our diets are when compared to the diet of our parents and grandparents. Of note, most of the causes of death around 1900 were from pathogenic diseases, meaning bacteria, viruses, or parasites. Some of the most common causes in the day were pneumonia, flu, TB, and gastro-intestinal infections that caused severe diarrhea. Compare that to today's major causes of death: chronic/inflammatory diseases such as heart disease, cancer, and cerebrovascular disease, creating huge at-risk populations with the COVID-19 pandemic.

**Causes of Death—US**
per 100,000

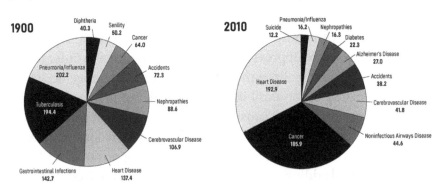

Figure 13.1. Since the introduction of edible seed oils to our diet, many deaths today are due to chronic/inflammatory diseases as compared to 100–150 years ago when pathogenic (bacterial) diseases were the leading cause of death.

## Obesity Epidemic

We can see, too, how the rate of obesity has changed dramatically during this same time period. In the early twentieth century, obesity was rare; in 1960, rates were already up 13 to 14%, but, by 1999, the obesity rates had risen to over 30%. According to data from the Centers for Disease Control, the obesity rate reached 42% in 2017-2018 and 29 out of 50 states projected to have more than 50% of their population struggling with obesity.[1] These staggering statistics show us that obesity is at epidemic proportions and is likely the biggest healthcare crisis we are experiencing at the present time, especially brought to light with the COVID-19 pandemic.

We only need to look back at images from the 1950s of young adults compared to today's young adults to see how things have changed—and when we're young, we're supposed to be at our healthiest!

## Where We Were to Where We Are

We so often hear that it's the significant increase in the amount of sugar we are consuming that is creating the obesity problem. However, the biggest change in our diet over the years is not from sugar consumption but from the unbelievable increase in vegetable and seed oil consumption. According to Dr. Chris Knobbe's research, between 1860 and 1909, we consumed an average of 2 g of vegetable oil per day. By 2010, we were consuming 80 g/day. This represents a 4,000% increase! That comes to an average of 720 calories of our recommended 2,000 calorie-a-day goal just from vegetable and/or seed oil; or, in other words, 36% of our daily calories.[2] If we look at just omega-6 consumption, in 1865 we consumed an average of 2.2 g of omega-6 per day, which was less than 1% of our total calories. In 1909, consumption of omega-6 had risen to 4.84 g/day, which then equaled about 2% of daily caloric intake. By 1999, it was up to 18 g/day, which was about 7% of the daily caloric intake. Data from 2008 show that we were consuming approximately 29 g/day of omega-6, which translates to approximately 11.8% of our daily caloric intake. The numbers from 2008 show 12 times more omega-6 consumption in our daily diets than in 1865.[3]

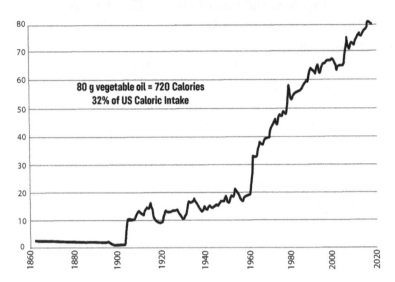

## Total Vegetable Oil Consumption in the US

80 g vegetable oil = 720 Calories
32% of US Caloric Intake

Figure 13.2. Between 1909 and 2010, there was a 4,000% increase of our daily consumption of vegetable and seed oil. That's 80 g/day, accounting for an average of 720 calories of our recommended 2,000 calories/day.

The vegetable oils are the main source of omega-6 fatty acids in our diet. The first oil marketed was cotton seed oil in 1865. In 1865, our primary sources of fat were from butter, lard, and beef tallow. The percentage of omega-6 in butter at that time was 1%; in lard and beef tallow, the percentage of omega-6 was 2%. These numbers change depending on what the animal eats. Grass-fed animals will have less omega-6 content than grain fed animals. Most animals nowadays are grain-fed and will, therefore, have a higher omega-6 content; in fact, these days, lard is no longer considered a saturated fat, since it is coming from pigs that are eating diets primarily composed of grains.

Oils that we eat get stored in our cells. This has changed dramatically through the years. Studies of tissue biopsies have shown that adipose tissue (connective tissue in which fat is stored) from 1959 contained 9.1% omega-6 (*linoleic acid*), compared with 21.5% omega-6 tissue biopsies from 2008.[*]

This is a huge amount when compared to cultures that eat a non-processed food diet like the Tokelauans, a tribal culture from an island in the South Pacific. When their tissue samples were tested in 1968, their adipose tissue contained only 3.8% omega-6.[5]

---

### Takeaways from Chapter 13

1. Historically, the intake of PUFA across societies was very low; there were no seed oils in our diet until the last 150 years.

2. The biggest change in our diet over the years is not from sugar consumption but from the unbelievable increase in vegetable and seed oil consumption.

3. PUFA is our number one health—and weight loss—enemy! PUFAs are found in seed and vegetable oils and fish oil; both omega-3 and omega-6—which are thought to be healthy fats—are actually pro-inflammatory!

---

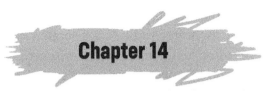

# Chapter 14

# Omega-6 versus Omega-3: Which One is Worse?

So, we can see that omega-6 invites inflammation throughout the body, but what about omega-3? Isn't it supposed to be anti-inflammatory, and isn't it supposed to be good for us? A question to ask is how people stayed healthy in the past without fish oil capsules. Let's look at the facts about omega-3.[1]

The story line is that omega-3 fats are "anti-inflammatory," which is partially true, but only when compared to omega-6 fats. Omega-3 fats still cause inflammation, just less so than that of the omega-6 fats.[2] So why has omega-3 become so popular recently? One possible reason is that companies have found a way to take a byproduct of fish processing that used to be discarded and turn this former wasted product into a substantial revenue stream. And it has now become a huge money maker: estimates suggest that by the year 2026, the fish oil market will make over $5 billion in sales of omega-3 fish oil products.[3] Another question to ask would be, is the popularity of the omega-3 fish oil product the cause of more inflammation in our population?

Let's look at why omega-6 and omega-3 are so problematic.

Omega-3 contains alpha-linolenic acid, EPA, and DHA, all of which act like anti-freeze in cold-water fish. It stays liquid at cold temperatures, which is why you can store it in the refrigerator, and it doesn't solidify like saturated fats such as coconut oil or butter. This makes sense because if it did solidify, the cold-water fish would get stiff and would be unable to swim, move, or function. Staying liquid at low temperatures is great for fish, but at room temperature, omega-3 will spontaneously oxidize, making it extremely unstable, especially in your body, where it is 98.6 degrees.

This oxidation creates free radicals that damage lipid mitochondrial membranes throughout the body.[4] These free radicals are also doing damage to other cellular molecules such as proteins and DNA. Studies show that these free radicals accelerate vascular aging by at least ten years, leading to inflammation, increased hardening of arteries, increased cardio-vascular disease, and increased cancer.[5] While omega-3 has become known for its anti-inflammatory properties, what people often don't talk about is the way in which it can actually contribute to inflammation throughout the body.

The reason that people talk about omega-3 as an anti-inflammatory compound is that in competing for the same enzymes that convert omega-6 into inflammatory end products, it minimizes the damage that these end products can have on the cell.[6] Omega-3 suppresses some parts of the immune system that produce inflammation,[7] which seems to be a good thing, but the suppression of B cells and T cells can be problematic, since they are important players in mounting the necessary immune response against bacteria, viruses, and cancers.[8]

Indeed, omega-3 has been shown to be effective in controlling some autoimmune conditions such as autoimmune hepatitis and asthma. This may all seem like good news in the short term, but, in the long term, it's a terrible trade-off and comes at a hefty price.

Another problem with omega-3 is that when it's metabolized, it can cause a build-up of fatty compounds in the liver, leading to NAFLD (non-alcoholic fatty liver disease)—this is, unfortunately, fairly prevalent in our society today. This is not a benign condition, as it is negatively impacting our liver function, associated with loss of proper liver function over time.[9]

---

### Takeaways from Chapter 14

1. Omega-6 (found in seed/vegetable oils) and Omega-3 (found in fish oil) are both inflammatory.

2. Omega-3 suppresses the immune system.

3. When omega-3 is metabolized, it can cause a buildup of fatty compounds in the liver, leading to a condition known as non-alcoholic fatty liver disease (NAFLD).

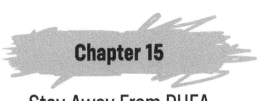

# Chapter 15

# Stay Away From PUFA

You may be asking, "So what is the big deal if our cells contain more PUFA?" The reason it is such an important issue is when the cells contain more PUFA, then the cell membranes contain more of this same omega-6. Through a fairly complex biochemical reaction involving damage to a substance known as *cardiolipin*, the cell's capacity for energy production is greatly reduced with increased omega-6 concentrations. Damaging cardiolipin also leads to insulin resistance and impaired fat metabolism. All of this makes weight loss more difficult. In addition, damaging cardiolipin causes damage to the cells' DNA, which then leads certain cells to multiply out of control—this is what eventually causes cancer. Damaging cardiolipin even affects the heart, which can then lead to heart failure. It also leads to increased production of free radicals, and as we noted in the prior chapter, these do a lot of damage throughout the body.[1] Specifically, in the heart, free radicals damage the mini power plants of the heart cells—the mitochondria. In one four-week experiment with rats that were fed rat chow with 20% safflower oil (PUFA) added to their diet, there was a 32% reduction in cardiac output. This means that there was heart damage after just four weeks with less PUFA in their diet comparitively than there is in the diet of the average American.[2]

Looking at the graph below (Fig 15.1), you can see that any amount of PUFA lowers the heart's ability to pump.

## What PUFA Does To The Body

The first problem with unsaturated fats is because they are unstable, they degrade quickly, and, when they do, they release free radicals that can cause significant damage to the cell's DNA. Free radical generation occurs when these oils are exposed to oxygen, heat, and/or

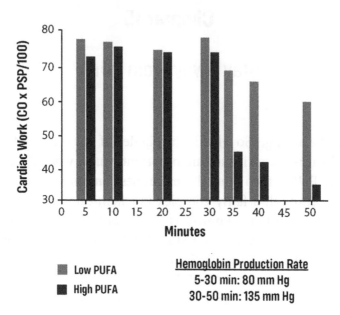

**High and Low PUFA Diet**

Figure 15.1. Any amount of PUFA in your diet lowers your cardiac output. However, with a high PUFA diet, your heart pumps significantly less, causing damage.

light. These types of oils were used in paint thinners and varnishes in the late 1800s and early 1900s because of their quick-drying qualities due to their rapid oxidation. This was before petroleum products took their place. For this reason, many edible vegetable and seed oils are in dark-colored bottles, and it is advised to store them in cool, dark places. The problem with how easily these oils can produce free radicals when exposed to oxygen, heat, and/or light is that when you consume them, you have oxygen and heat inside of you, which causes this free radical generation process to happen inside your body almost immediately.

So, let's go into greater detail about where PUFA causes problems and why it's so unhealthy.

**PUFA inhibits the thyroid gland and prevents it from producing thyroid hormone.** As we talked about in Chapter 6, thyroid hormone is the master hormone of the body and the main hormonal determinant of our metabolism. If we have enough thyroid hormone in circulation, we will have a fast metabolism, and, if we are deficient in thyroid hormone, we'll have a slow metabolism. With a slow metabolism, the body will burn fewer calories. Some people then will decrease their caloric intake attempting to lose the weight gained from a slowing metabolism; however, as mentioned earlier, fewer calories mean even fewer thyroid hormones and even slower metabolism.

**PUFA also blocks thyroid hormone from acting on the cell.** Hormones like the thyroid hormone create reactions by fitting into receptors, which then create a certain chemical reaction from the cell. It is exactly like a key fitting into a lock that we spoke of earlier. If the correct key fits, it opens the lock, and, if it is the wrong key, the lock won't open. If the wrong key is in the lock, then you can't put the right key in because the lock is blocked.

This is what happens when we talk about receptors being blocked or inhibited. PUFA inhibits the thyroid hormones from working at the receptor. When this happens, we call it a functional thyroid deficiency since we may have enough thyroid hormones circulating throughout the body, but what thyroid hormones we have are not able to function at the cell. That has the same outcome as if you are low on thyroid hormone. So that means that we can go to the doctor with all the symptoms of low thyroid-like fatigue, weight gain, depression, hair loss, low libido, and so on. Your healthcare provider does the blood test and says, "Everything looks good." As we talked about in Chapter 6, your healthcare provider may likely tell you, "You just need to eat less and workout more" to compensate for any weight gain resulting from slowed metabolism. Based on what we have just been illustrating, this is the worst thing you can do for your metabolism at this point.

**PUFA is the main driver of inflammation.** Omega-6 (linoleic acid) is the precursor to arachidonic acid, which is converted into multiple compounds that create inflammation throughout the body—namely, eicosanoids, prostaglandins, leukotrienes, and thromboxanes.

By the way, this is how NSAIDs like Advil (ibuprofen) and aspirin work to provide pain relief. They prevent arachidonic acid from being converted into prostaglandins and other inflammatory compounds by blocking the enzyme that allows this conversion.

The negative effects of arachidonic acid on our GI tract, our kidney, and our heart are substantial and hardly insignificant. Since

# Omega-6

## Linoleic Acid (LA)

## Arachidonic Acid (AA)

## Pro-Inflammatory:
Eicosanoids
Prostaglandins
Leukotrienes
Thromboxanes

Figure 15.2. Omega-6 (a linoleic acid) is the precursor to arachidonic acid, which is converted into multiple compounds that create inflammation throughout the body.

inflammation is the cause or a component of almost any disease, we can think of our number one goal as always keeping inflammation as low as possible. Instead of taking a medication to block inflammation, we say that it is much better not to consume the food(s) that create it!

**PUFA blocks energy production of the cell.** As we talked about earlier, every cell in the body produces energy. The generator for this energy is the mitochondria, which is the mini power plant of the cell. Earlier, when we were reviewing carbohydrates, we noted that making energy is primarily a three-step process. The last step in the process, the electron transport chain, is where most of the ATP energy is made. PUFA blocks a step in the electron transport chain by inhibiting a major enzyme called *cytochrome c oxidase*. This results in a significant decrease in the energy produced by the cells. If our cells are not making enough energy, they cannot work or function properly, which leads to many different diseases.[3]

**PUFA activates another enzyme, called the aromatase enzyme, responsible for converting testosterone into estrogen.** This is one of the main reasons men today have had a double-digit drop in testosterone since 1942, resulting in an average of 60% less testosterone than their grandfathers' generation. Remember, we discussed estrogen as a cause of cell proliferation, i.e., cancer, like prostate cancer. In addition, converting testosterone to estrogen in men causes muscle loss and "man boobs." Estrogen also causes excess fat storage and is another reason we have such an obesity problem among men today.

**PUFA inhibits the immune system.** Since PUFA increases cortisol, this will suppress the immune system.[4] We talked about this in Chapter 3 when we discussed effects of increased cortisol in creating stress response. In Europe, a mixture of omega-3 and omega-6 intravenous solution is actually given to organ transplant patients to suppress their immune system in order to prevent organ rejection.[5]

**Elevated PUFA drives metabolic syndrome.** It does so by increasing inflammation, which can lead to diabetes. It blocks the insulin receptor and gets in the way of the body's ability to oxidize glucose. This means your cells can no longer use glucose/sugar for an energy source, so it stays in the bloodstream, raising blood sugar levels to create inflammation throughout the body. Studies demonstrate that a diet high in unsaturated fats, like PUFA, is capable of predicting the development of diabetes years and even a decade before it happens.[6] And yet, a lot of people are still saying that PUFAs are healthy!

**PUFA may be the cause of inflammatory bowel disease and ulcerative colitis.** Ulcerative colitis is associated with increased dietary intake of fat omega-6, polyunsaturated fatty acids (PUFA).[7] This was suggested as far back as 2009 in a *BBC* news report: "A high intake of polyunsaturated fat may lead to inflammatory bowel disease."[8]

**PUFA plays a significant role in aging, one of its most detrimental aspects.** Most of us know of a person who has what is known as age spots, or we might even have them ourselves. They are sometimes called "liver spots." The technical term for these spots is *lipofuscin*, which means "dark fat," but they do not happen just on the skin. These are considered aging pigments and are found in the kidney, heart muscle, liver, adrenal glands, ganglion cells, and nerve cells. Lipofuscin is the outcome of a metabolic process that occurs when PUFA combines with iron. As we age, there is an accumulation of lipofuscin, which can lead to missteps in our protein metabolism and subsequent cell degeneration, ultimately leading to cell death. Studies show a causative effect of lipofuscin in neurodegenerative conditions such as Parkinson's Disease and Alzheimer's disease. Lipofuscin is a major factor in the biological aging of cells, ultimately leading to the gradual deterioration of function.[9]

**PUFA produces byproducts called aldehydes.** These are toxic substances that also create free radicals that damage the cell's function and its DNA. The aldehydes are cytotoxic, carcinogenic, atherogenic, and obesogenic. One of the most damaging kind of aldehydes found in PUFA is called acrolein; it is the simplest of the unsaturated aldehydes. Acrolein causes the burnt fat odor we smell when we cook with seed/vegetable oils. Acrolein is also known to be one of the main substances that causes lung cancer from smoking cigarettes. The amount of acrolein in a large order of french fries is equal to seventeen to twenty-six cigarettes, depending on the type and on the content of acrolein. This means that if you were to eat a regular order of french fries, or even a bag of potato chips, every day, it would be as bad for you as if you were smoking a pack of cigarettes a day.[10]

## Where PUFA Damage Happens and How It Contributes to Weight Gain

When we talk about the damage that PUFA does to cells and hormones, so often we're unaware of the immediate damage at the cellular level. But there is one result that we can all notice, and that is the effect that PUFA has on weight gain in modern society. One study, a three-week experiment using a high-fat diet in three groups of mice, shows the fat-gaining effects of omega-6. Each group received the same number of calories and the same amount of protein, carbohydrates, and fat. The only thing that was different within each group was the amount of omega-6 (PUFA) in the diet.[11]

One group's fat content was from beef tallow and linseed oil, which contained 4.4% omega-6; a second group was fed olive oil and linseed oil, which contained 7.7% omega-6; and a third group was fed safflower oil and linseed oil, which contained 36.6% omega-6. The findings were astonishing. The beef fat group gained 72 g, equivalent to a 27.6% weight gain from their initial starting weight; the olive oil group gained 90 g—or a 37.2% weight gain—from their initial starting weight; and the safflower group gained 116 g, or an amazing

43.2% weight gain, from their initial starting weight. This would be the equivalent of a person weighing 150 pounds gaining 65 pounds over a period of just a few months with a similar safflower oil and linseed oil diet! Remember that all three groups of mice ate the same calories and the same amount of protein, carbs, and fat in the three weeks of the study. The beef fat group did gain a smaller amount of weight by comparison, but their diet also included linseed oil. If their diet were beef fat alone, the omega-6 content would have been reduced to 1.4%, or a third of what was given in the study, and their overall weight gain would have been minimal. The study shows that keeping the calories the same and increasing only the omega-6 content increases weight gain by 43%.

To look at it another way, the beef tallow/beef fat group and the olive oil group had a much lower body fat percentage than the linseed oil/safflower oil group—i.e., 10.3%, 15.2%, and a staggering 54.5% body fat respectively.[12] And keep in mind that this occurred in these mice in only three weeks!

## We've Known About PUFA and its Harmful Effects for Many Years

The knowledge of how detrimental PUFA is goes back to as early as 1918, and maybe even before. Dr. Elmer McCollum, PhD, a biochemist and one of the first experts on diet and nutrition, wrote about this in his 1918 book *The Newer Knowledge of Nutrition*.[13] He performed an experiment with two groups of rats, in which he gave them both an identical diet, except one group was given 1.5% butter fat and the other group was given 5% bleached cottonseed oil (PUFA). The rats that were given the butter fat grew to normal size and lived on average of 1,020 days. The rats that were given cottonseed oil grew to only 60% of their normal size and lived only an average of 555 days, just a little over half as long as the rats eating the butter fat diet. These rats also suffered hair loss and emaciation. This suggests a fat-soluble vitamin deficiency.[14]

Another study in 2015, much more recent, was conducted over thirty-two weeks. This study used three groups of rats, all fed the same number of calories, with a diet that included 40% fat. The only difference among the three groups was the source of the fat in their diet. The control group was fed rat chow containing 1.2% linoleic oil (omega-6, PUFA); the second group was fed soybean oil, containing 2.2% linoleic oil; and the third group was fed soybean oil, containing 10% linoleic oil. After thirty-two weeks, the control group weighed 31 g. The second group fed with the 2.2% linoleic oil weighed 39 g, and the third group fed with 10% linoleic oil weighed 49 g. This last group had a 58% weight increase over the control group in the 32-week period. This would be equivalent to a person weighing 140 pounds gaining 71 pounds after eating this diet for 32 weeks.[15]

## Is PUFA Really An EFA?

With all the above said, PUFA has been deemed to be an essential fatty acid (EFA), meaning we must get it from our diet. This terminology came about in the 1930s where experiments were done with rats that were fed an essential fatty acid-deficient diet. Over time, the rats developed skin conditions that were reversed when they were fed EFAs.[16] This was a time when little was understood about certain vitamins. Subsequent studies demonstrated that when vitamin B6 was added to the diet, the skin condition symptoms improved. Therefore, it was determined that there was a need for more B vitamins in the diet to offset increased metabolism, which was a direct result of a diet without EFAs.

Now, as we're talking about the detrimental effects of PUFA, it is highly debatable whether we need EFAs at all or whether we might just need them in small amounts. Even proponents of EFAs agree that small amounts would be sufficient to meet all our body's needs. In fact, healthy traditional cultures consume little EFA. Studies done within these groups show daily linolenic acid (omega-6) consumption in the amounts of approximately 0.6–1.7 g/day versus our society's 40 g/day—and none of their EFA is from seed oils. These people are extremely healthy and appear to age without obesity, heart disease, or diabetes.[17]

Even if we try to avoid PUFA altogether, we easily get more than a sufficient amount of daily omega-3 and omega-6 in the diet. There is PUFA in all fat, even the most saturated fats; there is PUFA in meat, in eggs, and in dairy. Each of these sources contain more than a sufficient amount—in fact, more EFA than we will ever need. And this does not account for the abundance of PUFA in fish, grains, nuts, and seeds. With all of this in mind, it is difficult to stay below 4 g/day, even when making a determined effort.

Let's summarize the reasons to not eat a high PUFA diet.

- It inhibits thyroid hormone production and thyroid gland function.
- It is the main driver of systemic inflammation.
- It blocks energy production of ATP.
- It increases estrogen.
- It inhibits the immune system.
- It plays a main role in the development of metabolic syndrome and diabetes.
- It increases the stress response and levels of the primary stress hormone cortisol.
- It leads to inflammation of the intestines which in turn can lead to inflammatory bowel disease.
- And possibly most detrimental, it increases the aging of cells, which results in a significantly shorter life span.

## Takeaways from Chapter 15

1. PUFA is the main driver of inflammation.

2. PUFA blocks energy production within the body's cells, inhibiting both thyroid hormone production and thyroid gland function.

3. One of the most detrimental aspects of PUFA is the significant role it plays in advancing the body's aging process.

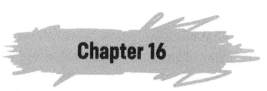

# Chapter 16

# The Good Fat—Saturated Fat

We have just talked about PUFA, the bad fat, but there is actually a good fat that is healthy, hormone balancing, and pro-metabolic. PUFA is the fat we don't want to eat. The fat that we want to eat more of is saturated fat (SFA). Remember from above, we talked about saturated fats as the types of fat that do not have any double bonds. Since they do not have double bonds, they are much less likely to produce the free radicals that can do an enormous amount of damage throughout the body. Also, having no double bonds, the chains of fatty acids are straight without any bends, which allows them to stack together tightly and become a solid. As we referenced earlier, there is an easy way to know if fats are saturated or not. SFA will remain solid at room temperature, and PUFA will liquefy at room temperature. For our purposes, any fat that is a solid at room temperature will be considered a saturated fat. (There are a few exceptions, like MCT [Medium Chain Triglyceride], and a few others, but they really are not part of the Diet Plan in this book.) For saturated fats in our Diet Plan, we are focusing on dairy fats, avocado oil, and coconut oil.

## Changing Our Minds About Saturated Fat

We know most people have heard at one time or another that saturated fat is bad for them, and that it will cause heart disease.[1] Research now shows this to be completely false; it may have been one of the most confusing pieces of advice given from the medical community about our health.[2] This information was based on poor science and more likely ulterior motives by food manufacturers for financial profit. What food manufacturers would benefit from telling people that cholesterol and saturated fat are bad for our health? From as far back as people can remember, up until the 1950s and 1960s, what most people ate for breakfast was bacon, eggs, and toast with butter. Then suddenly, these foods were now "bad," allowing cold cereals to become the mainstay of the American breakfast—which can now be seen by the full aisles of cereal in grocery stores.

Let's look at research showing some specific health benefits from eating saturated fat.

Researchers have been studying the benefits of saturated fats for many decades, and recently the mainstream media and medical community have begun to report its benefits. One such story was presented by *CNN News*, in 2017, on a study published in *The British Journal of Sports Medicine*. An excerpt from an editorial on the study is shown here:

> Three cardiologists say saturated fats do not clog arteries and the "clogged pipe" model of heart disease is "plain wrong." The authors wrote that "eating saturated fats is not associated with either coronary heart disease, ischemic stroke, type 2 diabetes, death from heart disease or early death in healthy adults," and "This idea that dietary saturated fats build up in the coronary arteries is complete unscientific nonsense," said Dr. Aseem Malhotra, first author of the controversial editorial and a consultant cardiologist at London's Lister Hospital, in an email to CNN.[3]

An example of the benefits of saturated fat is shown in a study done with mice that were fed a combination of soybean oil and canola oil for sixteen weeks. This diet caused significant heart damage to all of the mice. However, adding saturated fat to their diet dramatically reduced the damage.[4]

The prestigious *Journal of the American College of Cardiology* published an article in 2020 that states, "The recommendation to limit dietary saturated fatty acid (SFA) intake has persisted despite mounting evidence to the contrary. Most recent meta-analyses of randomized trials and observational studies found no beneficial effects of reducing SFA intake on cardiovascular disease (CVD) and total mortality, and instead found protective effects against stroke." The article went on to say that, "Whole-fat dairy, unprocessed meat, eggs, and dark chocolate are SFA-rich foods with a complex matrix that are not associated with increased risk of CVD. The totality of available evidence does not support further limiting the intake of such foods."[5]

This means you can go ahead and eat the foods that taste good, like ice cream and chocolate, and you don't necessarily have to worry so much about heart disease.

Dr. Ray Peat writes in his article "Fats, Functions & Malfunctions" that when a person is healthy or is still a child, the stress hormones adrenaline and cortisol are produced in essentially normal amounts, due to the consumption of free saturated fatty acids. These free saturated fatty acids block the production of excess adrenaline and cortisol. When a person eats a high PUFA diet, the stored fat is made up mainly of PUFA. The free fatty acids from PUFA are linoleic acid and arachidonic acid, which in turn stimulate the stress hormones, and this causes the release of more free fatty acids. This becomes a vicious cycle. Eating saturated fat actually decreases our stress response, and eating PUFA actually increases our stress response.[6] Saturated fatty acids have also been shown to improve immune system function and prevent tumor growth and metastasis.[7]

One of the most important effects of eating saturated fat is the protective effect that saturated fats have for the liver. Research shows that they can reverse alcohol-induced liver cell damage, and even fibrosis. This reversal can occur even if the person continues to ingest alcohol.[8]

A more real-world example is looking at groups of non-westernized cultures which obtain many of their calories from saturated fat. One such culture is the Maasai tribe of Tanzania, whose members eat a diet of 3,000 calories a day, a diet consisting mostly of meat, dairy, and blood. In their diet, they consume 66% of their calories as saturated fat. Studies showed that they had no obesity, and that heart disease was almost non-existent. Another such culture is the people who live on the Tokelau Islands in the South Pacific. Their diet consists of fish, starchy tubers, coconuts, and fruit, and they consume 48% of their calories from saturated fat. Neither group consumed any seed oils, and neither group suffered from obesity or heart disease.[9]

Another culture that eats a high-saturated-fat diet and lives to an old age are the Azerbaijans, a mountain people in the Middle East who eat high amounts of saturated fat and low amounts of polyunsaturated fat. Most of the fat in their diet comes from sheep fat, dairy, and meat, i.e., lamb and mutton. They consume little unsaturated fat. Their longevity in the 1981 census had 14,486 people over the age of 100 years—the equivalent of 48.3 people per 100,000. They also had many people in that group who were 120 years old.[10]

The other healthy fat that is fine to eat is MUFA, the monounsaturated fatty acid. These are the oils that have only one double bond. This fat does not oxidize as quickly, nor does it have the same damaging free radical effects as PUFA. The two most common types of MUFA are olive oil and avocado oil. Most people have heard of the benefits of the Mediterranean diet. One of the important components of the Mediterranean diet is olive oil.

---

## Takeaways from Chapter 16

1. PUFA is bad fat, but saturated fats are good fats and necessary for overall optimal health and wellness. They have been shown to improve our immune system and prevent tumor growth and metastasis.

2. Incorporating saturated fats into the daily diet has been controversial, but data show no beneficial effects from limiting their intake in our daily diet.

3. MUFAs are another healthy fat; the two most common types are avocado oil and olive oil, which is one of the important components of the Mediterranean diet.

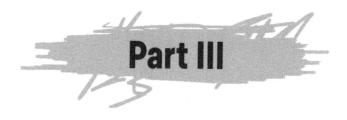

# Part III

## The Plan

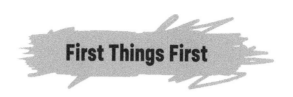

# First Things First

We are going to work on making some significant lifestyle changes. This means that we are going to take action! The great news is we can take some small actions and get big results. Everyone has a different state of current health, different genes, unique backgrounds, and different environments. So, on the road to better health and optimal performance, we have to start from where we are. This also means that there is not one plan that is right for everyone. It is actually for this reason that so many health programs and diets fail. They give you a list of foods, supplements, and exercises that may be right or wrong for you, and if you do not "succeed," they leave you believing it's your fault. That is definitely not how this plan works. There are certain "laws" that we will need to follow, but once we follow the major rules, then we are able to determine which method is right for us.

So now let's get going. The plan is comprehensive and addresses all of the following. There is no expectation that you need to do all of these in order to start feeling better.

- diet
- supplements
- sleep
- exercise
- mindfulness/meditation

With this plan, we will improve our overall health and achieve our optimal daily energy, no matter what age!

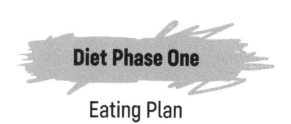

# Diet Phase One

## Eating Plan

### The Number One Thing—No PUFA!

Some patients ask us, "If you could tell me only one thing to do to make me better, what is it?" We always tell them that diet and nutrition have many parts, but, if we are limited to just one thing they can do to dramatically improve their health, it would be to eliminate PUFA from their diet.[1]

Eliminating PUFA from one's diet takes effort, but the health benefits are enormous. Though the benefits take a little time to notice, most people start to feel better within three weeks. The longer you avoid polyunsaturated fats, the greater the effect on your health. Remember that there is no magic pill for health. Just like working out to stay in shape, we have to make it a lifestyle and not think of it as a short-term solution. The benefits of eliminating PUFA from our diet are significant:

- feeling more energetic
- lowering blood sugar
- decreasing inflammation
- developing a healthier GI tract
- creating a faster metabolism
- improving the immune system
- balancing out the hormones

So, the first thing to do to avoid PUFA is to get rid of all the seed oils in your house, including these:

- canola oil (grape seed)
- corn oil
- safflower oil
- soybean oil
- sunflower oil

- cottonseed oil
- peanut oil
- palm oil
- flaxseed oil
- lard (high in PUFA due to grain-fed pigs)

We want to read labels and ask questions, donating or throwing out all foods processed with seed oils as shown in the list above.

Once we cut out the PUFA, there are a few restrictions. We will still eat meat, fish, dairy, vegetables, and fruit, but only those cooked or processed without any of the seed oils. We want to try to cook primarily with olive oil, coconut oil, beef tallow, butter, or avocado oil.

We always say it's better to prepare our food at home, if we can, but that may not work for many of us due to work schedules and time.

Now that you know you need to stay away from PUFA, what do you do? We will try to make it easy for you to leave polyunsaturated fats behind and start to include more saturated fats in your diet.

The safe oils we can use to replace PUFA are saturated animal fats, dairy fats, and monounsaturated fats including the following:

- butter
- coconut oil
- avocado oil (MUFA)
- beef tallow
- olive oil[2]

When you start reading the ingredients on all packaged foods, you might notice that almost every packaged food will contain an abundance of PUFA. In fact, once you start reading the ingredients, you will be amazed at how many things are made or processed with polyunsaturated fat. There is also a common belief that everything in organic grocery stores like Whole Foods, Sprouts, or Natural Grocers will be healthy, but it is just not true. In fact, most things in those stores are still loaded with some type of seed oil. Manufacturers make these oils sound healthy because they will list them as organic canola, organic soy, or organic corn oil, but "organic" in no way makes these oils healthy. Even the food in the buffet areas is loaded with canola oil and/or soybean oil. The food manufacturers have wised up to the fact that people are now trying to avoid PUFA, so they have tried to disguise it. An example is the many salad dressings and mayonnaises that will say they are made with avocado oil or with olive oil—but, when you read the ingredients on the label, canola oil or soybean oil is still listed as one of the top ingredients.

So, now you're reading labels and switching out PUFA for the unsaturated fats—what's next to achieve your optimum health?

The best advice we have heard was from Jack LaLanne. He was known as the "Original Health Nut." He was born in 1914 and died in 2011 at the age of ninety-seven years. He credited his diet of healthy non-processed foods and natural juices for taking him from an unhealthy teenager to a healthy adult. LaLanne often said he had never been sick a day in his adult life. His first daily show on television in the 1950s taught women how to work out at home. When we show his picture at seminars, older adults will say they remember his show; younger adults know him as the "Juice Man." When asked what the perfect diet was, LaLanne would say, "Don't eat anything in a package."[3]

Since many of us dine out, there are foods that we need to put on the "Do Not Eat" list. This means all fried foods unless the food is fried in a saturated fat like beef tallow or duck fat. Although this is pretty uncommon, there are a few restaurants that do this—Outback Steakhouse, for one. Of course, that does mean no french fries, no chicken fingers, and no corn chips at the Mexican restaurants. These are some of the biggest offenders! Another item that we don't typically think about as a PUFA is salad dressing. If it is made with olive oil, many times, the olive oil is a counterfeit made with canola oil. Olive oil counterfeits have been a big problem in the food industry.

So, what are the replacement foods? One suggestion is if you like to eat a lot of salads when you dine out, then plan to bring your own dressing or oils in a small container, or you can just ask the restaurant for olive oil and vinegar. Most restaurants will be able to provide them. If you are going to a Mexican restaurant, you can bring your own chips that are cooked with olive or avocado oil. It's better to avoid them altogether, but the good news is you can eat the flour or corn tortillas with butter in the place of chips. Also, it's a good idea to try to eat at restaurants that are "farm to table." Most of the time, these restaurants cook with healthier oils.

Avoiding PUFA doesn't mean you have to give up everything that is enjoyable. Remember, you can eat foods that contain saturated fats and sugar. If you want potato chips, look for the ones made with olive, avocado, or coconut oils. The same goes for all packaged items. It takes some searching, but most items you can find made with the good fats. If you want desserts, many of the premium brands of ice cream are made without PUFA. You can also find baked goods like pies, cookies, and croissants made with butter instead of oils.

## Eat Enough Calories

It may seem strange that we start talking about a diet by saying you must "eat enough." Though you would think it goes without saying that we should eat enough to be healthy, that is one of the biggest mistakes we see people make. This is especially true with people who diet or who are so busy they do not take time to eat. We also see undereating with people who are under stress and are not "hungry." They don't often feel like eating because they are running on stress hormones of cortisol, adrenaline, and caffeine, all of which tend to suppress appetite. This makes sense when compared to people who take ADHD medications like Adderall or Ritalin. They never want to eat and don't have much of an appetite. You know the type who seem to just live on coffee—we have actually had people come to us who drink three pots of coffee a day and take Adderall. Remember that we need to eat to produce energy, and, if we're not, then it's the stress hormones that are giving us the energy in an unhealthy way, by wasting our muscles as fuel. That's definitely the last thing we're going for!

When we discuss eating habits with people, they often respond that they understand, but they also acknowledge that it doesn't make sense to them that they need to eat more to lose the weight. We have all been indoctrinated that wanting to lose weight means cutting the calories, but this is exactly what puts us back on the merry-go-round of weight gain/weight loss and contributes to the majority of yo-yo dieters' stubborn weight gain and failed efforts at weight loss. Though this tends to be much more prominent in women, we see it with both men and women. We are not picking on women, but our culture has placed a high value on women looking a certain way, like the women we have seen in movies, on television, and on magazine covers that have been photoshopped. It was only more recently that ads, movies, and television shows have begun to feature women who are not underweight.

Women will come in eating under 900 calories per day, which is essentially a starvation diet. They come in suffering with symptoms of fatigue, depression, anxiety, inability to sleep, hormonal issues, and problems with their monthly cycle. Many times, most of this will resolve itself when we just increase their calories to give their bodies enough energy to get them out of the stress mode of starvation. These patients have been living on fat-free yogurt and carrot sticks for their daily meals. Once a woman starts eating real food with sufficient calories, she feels like a different person. Though she may gain some weight at the beginning until the metabolism returns to normal, this is the only real way to heal.

## Setting Up Your Caloric Intake

Here are a few common questions we hear when talking about how to eat: "How many proteins, carbs, and fat carbs should I eat?" "Should I follow a low-carb diet?" "Is being a vegetarian healthy?"

Let's talk about how many proteins, carbs, and fats you should eat. First, there is not a "one-size-fits-all" answer. It will depend on your unique situation. How active are you? Do you have a slow or fast metabolism? Do you have a problem with insulin resistance? Are your hormones balanced? What we can talk about are some general rules that will apply to all of us, namely that we should incorporate all three macronutrients—proteins, fats, and carbs—into our daily diet. Choosing the right type of fats and carbs, in addition to the right amounts, is crucial to supplying the body with everything it needs for optimal performance.

There are cultures from around the world that stay healthy eating a wide variety of proteins, carbs, and fats.

An example of this is the Masai tribe we discussed previously. They actually eat a high-fat diet, stay healthy, and live long lives. On the opposite extreme, there are the Okinawans, who are also long-lived and who tend to be the healthiest people on the planet. They have a diet ratio of 10:1 carbohydrate to protein. Their diet consists of 85% carbohydrates. This high-carbohydrate, low- protein, low-fat diet is just the opposite of what the low-carb, high-fat/protein advocates say.[4]

## How Much Protein?

When it comes to protein, the range is anywhere between 10 and 35% of our daily caloric intake. For example, if we're eating 2,000 calories a day, that will mean anywhere from 200–700 calories would be coming from protein. One gram of protein is equal to 4 calories, so that would be 50–175 g of protein per day with a 2,000 calorie diet. Some studies show the average adult needs at least 0.8 grams of protein per kilogram of body weight to prevent protein deficiency.[5] So, if a person weighs 160 pounds, that means they would need at least 58 gms of protein per day. If you are an athlete, or if you're lifting weights and body building, you may actually need up to 1.4–2.0 grams of protein per kilogram of body weight. Right now, the average American 19–30 years old is eating 91 +/- 22 g of protein a day. High-protein diets can have a person eating up to several hundred grams of protein a day. This can cause significant health problems, if consuming too many grams of protein without adequate amounts of fats and carbohydrates in the diet.

Unlike the other macronutrients, you can get too much protein. Once you get above 35% of your calories from protein, the excess amino acids will be converted to ammonia. Normally, the ammonia is converted to urea and excreted through the kidneys. When there is excess protein, the body's ability to excrete the ammonia is limited, and the body will have a buildup of ammonia, which is toxic to our nervous system.

This problem was seen in the early frontier days of the US. In winter, when game was scarce, the most common food available was rabbits. Since rabbits have extraordinarily little fat, these settlers were eating a diet that was predominantly protein. They would often develop a condition called "Rabbit Wasting Disease." The symptoms would include nausea, diarrhea, nervous system failure, and even death, all of which can happen in as little as two weeks. This means that people who are eating a high-protein/low-carb diet must make sure to incorporate enough fat in their diet to balance out the high-protein intake.[6]

Here are some examples of the protein content of meats, such as beef, pork, chicken, turkey, and fish:

- One ounce of beef, turkey, pork, chicken, turkey, or fish: each is roughly equivalent to 7 g. If you ate four ounces of meat or fish, that would equal roughly 28 g of protein.
- One egg equals 6 g of protein.

A good rule of thumb is to include at least four ounces of protein with each meal.

Collagen is one of the best sources of protein. Collagen is the most abundant protein in our bodies. It's the main building block for the connective tissue of the skin, cartilage, and tendons. Collagen has known health benefits like improving and strengthening hair, skin, and nails. Also, collagen is known to decrease joint pain and improve GI health, brain function, and sleep.

One of the components that make collagen so good for you is the amino acid *glycine*. You see in America that our culture has eliminated most organ and other animal parts from the daily diet, except for muscle meat. Muscle meat is high in the amino acids *tryptophan* and *methionine*, but it is deficient in glycine. This means that most people are deficient in glycine, which we will discuss in greater detail in the supplements section.

## How Many Carbohydrates?

This is the macronutrient that is the latest culprit for all of the medical and health woes of modern society, per the medical community. But, hopefully, we have demonstrated throughout this book that it's actually the wrong kind of fat—i.e., polyunsaturated fats—and the increased stress response that comes with the release of free fatty acids blocking the cells' use of glucose, which is really the main driver of most of our health problems in the US. In fact, to our knowledge, there has never been a culture throughout history that has voluntarily given up consuming carbohydrates if they were available. Of course, there are cultures that during times of scarcity may not have had access to them, such as the Innuits in the far north.

What is the right amount of carbohydrates in our daily diet? Some people feel great with 85% of their calories coming from carbs, and others feel better with only 33% of their calories coming from carbs. We recommend not going below 150 g/day—this is equivalent to approximately two to three servings of fruit per day, and one to two servings of starches, like potatoes and rice. If you go lower than 40–60 g/day of carbohydrates, your body will have to start using free fatty acids and ketone bodies for fuel (we talked about this earlier in Part One). Even though this sounds like a good thing, in a moment we will talk about why it's not. Some people who do not "do well" with carbs—meaning they feel bloated, fatigued, depressed, or have a feeling of cold/flu symptoms—are usually suffering from either a food intolerance or increased endotoxin from the large or small intestine. We covered this in great detail in Chapter 8 on GI health, and we will be talking about this more in the next section, which focuses on building the right microbiome.

For now, don't be afraid to eat carbs. It is fine to eat fruit, vegetables, and starches daily. Now this is the time when many people will ask, "Do you need to eliminate sugar entirely?" Some will say they have heard that sugar is the "root of all evil" and the reason why many people develop diabetes. While we are not advocating eating all your calories from sugar—namely, because it's devoid of nutrients—sugar is not the actual cause of insulin resistance, as we stated in detail in Chapter 5. Research shows that the cause actually involves more free fatty acids and the subsequent activation of the cortisol stress response.[7]

When people talk about how addictive sugary foods are (especially if we use the example of a donut or a bag of chocolate candy), people will always mention the sugar. No one ever talks about the PUFA that the donut is fried in or the seed oils that are used in processing the chocolate candies. If it were the sugar and not the fat that was addictive, people would just sit around and eat bags of sugar—it would be cheaper.

## How Much Fat?

As we discussed previously, we do not have to limit fat; we just need to eat the right kind of fat. Now that we know to eliminate polyunsaturated fat (PUFA), we really do not have to fear the saturated fats or the monounsaturated fats. This allows us to eat a great variety of food. We can eat butter and anything made with or cooked in coconut oil, olive oil and/or animal fats. It means we can eat eggs and even ribeye steaks without feeling guilty. We can eat ice cream and other desserts made with butter and cream. Some people will feel better eating 50% of their calories from fat, but some may do well with eating 10–15% of their calories from fat. If weight loss is your priority, or if you need to improve blood sugar levels, we recommend keeping fat calories on the lower end of the spectrum.

One of the largest nutrition studies of the last fifty years was a joint research study by the British through the University of Aberdeen in Scotland and the Chinese through the Chinese Academy of Sciences. They looked at two groups of mice, varying the amounts of proteins, carbs, and fats in their diets. They discovered that "an increased intake of dietary fats was found to drive obesity in mice more than an increase in protein or carbohydrates." They concluded that the least amount of weight gain was a diet composed of 10–20% fat calories.[8]

## Fad Diets

Many people ask if becoming a vegetarian is the best way to eat. For most people, it is not the healthiest diet. If someone is eating this way because of a religious or philosophical reason, then we respect their choices, and we want to meet people where they are. Most people that eat this way need to strongly supplement their diets, or, over a period of time, they will likely develop nutritional deficiencies such as fat-soluble vitamin deficiencies, vitamin B12 deficiencies, and protein deficiencies. This is not to say that a person can't be healthy with a vegetarian diet, but it just takes much more effort to prevent such effects. As mentioned, this may include taking a B12 supplement or other daily supplements in order to maintain optimal health. Eating a vegetarian diet for short periods of time may have more of a therapeutic effect, as opposed to trying to maintain a vegetarian diet for the long term.

What is meant by a therapeutic effect is that, in the short run, if a person has a deficiency of, for example, hydrochloric stomach acid, that person may have trouble digesting animal protein, and animal protein may make them feel sick until this is resolved. Another example is if a person has a virus or bacterial infection, it may take less energy to metabolize a vegetarian diet. Overall, eating animal protein that is humanely raised, and is hormone and antibiotic free, is much better for long term health. This is not to say that people must eat large amounts of animal protein, but a person can eat the minimum amount to meet their protein requirements.

One of the most common diet questions people ask is, "Should I eat a low-carb, ketogenic diet?" The ketogenic type of diet consists of eating low carb and generally high fat. After a few days of low carbs, the person depletes all the stored glycogen in the body and then produces ketone bodies, which can be used as an energy source. This diet is all the rage right now in the health community with biohackers and celebrities. Ketogenic diets have been touted as miracle diets that are the best for weight loss, lowering blood sugar, providing more energy, and the list goes on and on. Though the ketogenic diet is often touted as the latest and greatest diet, it is also one of the most debated subjects in nutrition today. For every research study that can be found about the benefits of eating this way, there is another study showing its negative effects.

When we speak of ketogenic (low carb) diets, one of the main benefits that people report is feeling much better at the beginning of the diet (less bloating, less swelling, and significant weight loss). They may also feel less fatigued and have fewer headaches, as well as fewer sugar and carb cravings. This is mainly because, when they eliminate carbohydrates from their diet, they have invariably reduced the soluble fiber and resistant starch that make their way to the large intestines to feed the Gram-negative bacteria. When diagnosing what is happening with the microbiome, this factor in itself is telling.

In the experience of working with thousands of people, we see that most people do not do well with their weight loss goals eating a ketogenic diet. We can always find exceptions of people doing well with any diet, of course, but overall, we so often find that those cases were really the exception rather than the rule. The first problem with this diet is that most people stay on a keto diet only for a short period of time. People will brag about how much weight they lost while they were eating low carbs and then turn around and say they gained all the weight back plus more when they attempted to return to normal eating. When asked why they stopped eating keto, they say it was just not sustainable, and they missed eating carbs. Many say they really missed eating fruit or bread so decided it was not worth it. Remember, we said that one of the most important criteria for a healthy diet is that it needs to be sustainable for the long term.

There is much conflicting research about whether eating a ketogenic diet will or will not control blood sugar. For some people, it will help, but, for many others, it can make blood sugar regulation problems much worse and even cause blood sugar to go out of control. We have had patients on a ketogenic diet that continue to have blood sugars running in the 200–300 range (normal is 110 or less), which is uncontrolled diabetes. Many people also complain that they would get "keto flu," a feeling like they are coming down with the flu; other people would say they were always fatigued while they were on the diet.

Although many people on the keto diet rave about the weight loss and lowered blood sugar, this finding is somewhat debatable in the scientific literature. One such study was published in the prestigious science journal Nature Metabolism in 2020. The study was conducted with rats, as with many studies, because it is difficult to test with humans. Results showed that reduction in weight loss and blood sugar happened only during the first one to two weeks of the keto diet. Most of the initial weight loss was due to water weight because, initially, the body is depleted of glycogen, and it is glycogen that holds fluid in the muscle.[9] When the glycogen is depleted, it acts like a diuretic, and the water leaves the muscle as glycogen levels are reduced.

This is a common complaint with people who eat a ketogenic diet—or any low-carb diet, for that matter. They see sometimes a twenty-pound weight loss within a few weeks, but then hit a plateau and can't lose any more weight. The person reacts by cutting carbs even more, and since they had what looked like "success" at the beginning, they are convinced that cutting back even more will result in more weight loss. When this does not produce any benefits, most will then give up in frustration and return to "normal" eating, which will put back the pounds lost (and plus some).

The same study also showed that after two to three months, the keto-fed mice gained significantly more weight compared to the mice that were fed regular rat chow, and the keto-fed mice also had higher fasting glucose levels. The researchers concluded, "Obesity on the keto-diet fed mice was driven by excessive whole-body fat accumulation including in the liver."[10] Ketogenic diets have also shown to increase NAFLD (non-alcoholic fatty liver disease) and can progress to cirrhosis, if untreated.[11]

With that said, some people may do well on a ketogenic diet and feel well eating this way, depending on their genetics and individual preferences, especially if they are younger and fairly fit. But, from working with thousands of people over time, the majority do not, and it's not generally sustainable. This diet, for them, creates a significant increase in the stress hormones; eventually, most of them gain weight after they stop eating this way.

A good description on how to eat would be a "paleo-with-a-twist diet," meaning a diet based on unprocessed, unpackaged (ideally, organic) foods, consisting of dairy, meats, and vegetables, including starchy root vegetables and plenty of fruit. If you want to eat a dessert a day, it's okay, as long as it doesn't contain PUFA. Do this for three weeks. Most people will see a noticeable improvement in just twenty-one days, but we really want to utilize this way of eating as a lifestyle, not just for the twenty-one days. For many people, twenty-one days will be enough to see noticeable improvements in their health; others who have more complicated health challenges or hormone imbalances will need to add our Phase Two GI Healing Plan in order to heal.

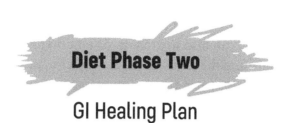

# Diet Phase Two

# GI Healing Plan

We talked earlier about the various functions/dysfunctions within the gastrointestinal (GI) system in Chapters 8 and 9. This part of the plan is for those who may be suffering with any type of ongoing gastrointestinal problem that doesn't involve bleeding. If you're bleeding, please see your medical doctor. Symptoms of a dysfunctional GI tract can range from bloating, indigestion, heartburn, gas, constipation, and/or loose bowels. This part of the eating plan is also for people whose GI problem(s) may be the cause of any one of a number of autoimmune conditions. You may not realize how problems with your GI tract may be affecting or causing these problems.

These types of autoimmune conditions include any of the following:
- chronic fatigue
- fibromyalgia
- Hashimoto's thyroid disease
- Grave's thyroiditis
- psoriasis
- rheumatoid arthritis
- eczema
- any other condition that has the body attacking itself

Even mood disorders such as depression and anxiety can be the result of chronic gastrointestinal problems.

But, the most common condition that people are suffering with (that is directly related to bowel issues) is weight gain. Remember (from Chapter 9 on endotoxin) that the body can become toxic from an overabundance of bacteria in the large or small intestine that can migrate through the intestinal wall and enter the bloodstream. These bacteria, once in the bloodstream, cause the body to mount a significant immune system response, often resulting in damaging inflammation throughout the body. Once the bacteria are in the bloodstream, they can also migrate to distant organs and body parts such as the brain and the joints. After the bacteria travel to these other areas of the body, they can trigger an overactivation of the immune response that mistakes the body for the bacteria and begins to kill off its own cells. All of this applies to endotoxin, as well. This is thought to be the basis for many autoimmune conditions.

To either eliminate "bad" bacterial overgrowth and/or endotoxin, or to prevent it from even happening, we must understand what the causes are and then work to eliminate them. This allows for healing of the intestinal tract and an optimal microbiome.

Some of the main contributors of chronic gastrointestinal distress are stress, inflammation, and certain types of foods. In our optimal health plan, we are always trying to find ways to reduce stress and inflammation; since one of the areas that we have the most control over is diet, we will focus on that.

Let's look at what we can do with our diet to achieve optimal GI health. We spoke in the last section about how stressful and inflamma-tory PUFA is to the body, and for that reason, that's the first thing we want to eliminate from our diet. For many people, this can and will result in drastic improvements in their intestinal health and may be enough, but, for many people, eliminating PUFA by itself, although necessary, will not be enough to resolve all of their problems. With ongoing autoimmune conditions, we will likely have to make more dietary changes in order to see the improvements.

To understand the dietary changes needed, we will have to go into more detail on why some foods may be problematic. The foods that have the biggest effect on general GI health are carbohydrates. Recall that carbs are the primary source of fuel for the body. The cells of the body convert glucose from the diet into ATP, which is the pri-mary energy source of the body. As we have talked about throughout the book, the body can use fat and ketone bodies as fuel, but if there is glucose around, the body will use that first. If the body runs out of glucose and its stored form of glycogen, the body will then burn fat and break down muscle and other tissues throughout the body, so they can convert protein into glucose. As we discussed earlier, this is done through the process of *gluconeogenesis*. This process of gluconeogenesis happens anytime we are under stress when cortisol and adrenaline—the stress hormones—are released.

## Four Main Types of Carbohydrates

We discussed earlier what carbohydrates are, but let's go into more detail on how they affect the GI system. For our purposes, we will classify and discuss four main types of carbohydrates:

- cellulose
- sugar
- starches
- fiber

## Cellulose

Cellulose is the structural component of the cell wall of green plants. It is non-digestible by humans but is a main food source for herbivores that have the digestive system to digest them, like horses and cows. So, for us humans, we really don't think about cellulose in the foods we eat. It doesn't really get counted among the carbs we take in, although it works really well as an insoluble fiber to help provide bulk to our GI waste products.

## Sugar and Starch

Often, carbs are divided into simple and complex carbs. Sugar is usually thought of as a simple carb, and starches are usually considered complex carbs. Sugars are further classified as *monosaccharides, disaccharides,* and *polysaccharides.*

Monosaccharide, as we learned earlier, means "one sugar." The main types of monosaccharides are glucose, fructose, and galactose. This means that all carbs that we eat, simple or complex, will eventually break down to one or more of these three monosaccharides.

Disaccharide means "two sugars." The three main disaccharides are sucrose, lactose, and maltose. Sucrose is table sugar—it has one molecule of glucose and one molecule of fructose connected together. Lactose is the sugar found in milk, and it is made up of one molecule of glucose and one molecule of galactose. Maltose is two molecules of glucose bound together, and it is found in starch.

Then we have polysaccharides, which are long chains of glucose molecules strung together, making up all the starches. Starches are found in grains, such as wheat and corn, and in vegetables such as white potatoes and sweet potatoes.

Simple sugars such as table sugar and fruit digest quickly in the stomach and the upper part of small intestines, so they shouldn't reach the large intestine. As a result, in ideal conditions, simple sugar will have no effect on the bacteria located there.

Starches can be classified as two different types, resistant and non-resistant. They behave differently.

Non-resistant starch, simply, is not resistant to digestion in the small intestine. As a result, it breaks down quickly in the small intestine before it gets to the large intestine. Resistant starch acts almost like fiber and is indigestible in the small intestine. So, it makes its way to the large intestine, where it is digested by the bacteria located there. This means resistant starch feeds both the good and the bad bacteria. There are some stated benefits of resistant starch in the large intestine. The bacteria ferment the starch, creating short-chain fatty acids that can be used as fuel by the body, and these fatty acids can lower blood sugar levels. Resistant starch is found in varying amounts in vegetables such as grains, legumes, and seeds. Although potatoes, green bananas, and other starchy foods are mostly made up of non-resistant starch, a small part of these starchy foods does contain resistant starch. Rice and potatoes cooked and then cooled will also create resistant starches. This is one reason a person can feel fine after eating fresh cooked potatoes or rice, but, if they are eaten the next day, it may create problematic GI symptoms like bloating, abdominal discomfort, and other symptoms we associate with endotoxin.

## Fiber

The next carbohydrate that is important for optimal GI health is fiber. We all "know" that fiber is good, right? But is this really true? Let's take a look at the different types of fiber. There are different ways to classify fibers. For our purpose, we will divide them into two different types, *soluble fiber* and *insoluble fiber*.

Fiber is indigestible by humans, but, if it is soluble fiber, it can be digested by bacteria once it travels to the large intestine. We don't have the enzymes necessary to digest the fiber, but the bacteria do. They digest the fiber through the process of fermentation, and just like with resistant starch, they create short chain fatty acids that can be used as fuel by the body; these fatty acids can lower blood sugar levels. This is one of the main benefits of taking in soluble fiber. Soluble fiber also adds bulk to the stool, and it lowers cholesterol. The negative effects of soluble fiber are the same as resistant starch: it feeds the bad bacteria as well as the good. Again, this can lead to increased bacterial growth of all the wrong types of gut bacteria; and if you have an inflamed intestinal wall, the bacteria (good and bad) can leak into the bloodstream, causing an immune system response. This immune system response will create increased inflammation throughout the body. And, of course, as bacterial growth increases, so does the endotoxin.

Insoluble fiber means that, like soluble fiber, humans cannot digest it, but, unlike soluble fiber, neither can the bacteria in the large intestine. What insoluble fiber is good for is preventing or alleviating constipation.[1] This is because it binds water and brings the water into the large intestine, making the stool softer. Also, insoluble fiber adds bulk to the stool, which makes bowel movements easier to pass. It also creates a feeling of fullness so it can prevent us from overeating.

Studies show that insoluble fiber speeds the rate of waste elimination in the colon, which reduces the exposure to toxins that are the by-products of digestion. Insoluble fiber also helps maintain an optimal pH level within the large intestine.

So, eating insoluble fiber is a starting place for developing better GI health if you have any of the conditions that we just mentioned. It's also an option if you don't feel as good as you should after eating a diet high in starchy or fibrous foods. Some people will describe it as just a feeling of being "off." This feeling starts within a short period of time after eating or can even begin a few days later. Why? Because it typically takes four to five hours for food to leave your stomach and then another three to six hours to get through the small intestine, until it finally gets to the large intestine, where it may take as many as thirty to forty hours to pass through. Therefore, it can be a few days before symptoms appear, as the bacteria multiply and the endotoxin increases.

This is one of the reasons correlating diet-related health problems to bowel issues is so difficult; most of the time, the response to eating certain foods is delayed. People often don't realize the response is tied to eating certain foods, since there's so much time between having eaten the problematic food and having the reaction. It's easy to know when you have an actual food allergy like a peanut allergy because you have an immediate, noticeable reaction that is often severe, unlike the insidious effects of bacteria and endotoxin.

The timing of when the symptoms happen can indicate where and what the problem is. Many people will come in and say that within three to four hours after eating, they feel bad. What this can tell us is that it is not their large intestine that is the source of the problem, but rather the stomach or the small intestine. Remember, it usually takes seven to ten hours for what you have eaten to reach the large intestine. If you feel symptoms immediately or within minutes after eating, the problem is usually coming from the stomach, i.e., a bacteria like H. pylori, an ulcer, or a food intolerance/allergy.

If the problems occur within four to six hours after eating, the source will more than likely be the small intestine—namely SIBO (small intestinal bacterial overgrowth). It's important to remember that the small intestine should be bacteria-free. Of course, if the problems are coming over ten hours after eating, now we are talking about the problem being further down the digestive tract, with the large intestine.

These reactions are not set in stone, of course, because everyone is different and gut motility can vary significantly from one person to another. Some people have extremely slow gut motility, and some people have relatively fast gut motility, and, as such, they may not fit the time frames noted above.

When symptoms happen within a short period of time, such as after eating fatty foods, this may indicate a bile deficiency from the gallbladder. Bile is needed to emulsify the fats you eat. If you don't feel well after eating protein, it could indicate a lack of hydrochloric acid in the stomach. Hydrochloric acid is needed to break down and digest protein such as meat.

In Phase Two, the GI Plan, we recommend eliminating all starches, fiber, and dairy for three days. For some people, this will sound easy enough, and, for other people, this will sound like climbing Mount Everest. But it's only for three days.

Since we do not want this to be a low-carb diet, we will replace the starchy carbs and fibrous food with fruit juices, no sugar added. The first three days, you can eat all the protein and fat (saturated and monounsaturated—olive oil, butter, avocado oil, coconut oil) that you want and drink fruit juices. Fruit juice should be pulp free, and, if you can get it, organic is always the best, with no sugar added. This can be orange juice, cranberry, cherry, apple, pineapple, grape, pomegranate, or any other juice you like. You can drink them individually or make a mix of different juices like orange juice, cranberry, and apple. The reason for using juices to start with is, for some people, even the fiber in some fruit can be a problem; however, the juice is readily absorbed before it makes it to the large intestine. Although there is no set amount for the day, ideally you should drink the juice at least four times a day to help keep the blood sugar fairly stable.

Remember, this is just a test to see how you react to starches and soluble fiber. If you feel better in any way, such as decreased bowel symptoms, decreased fatigue, better mood, or any of the aforementioned symptoms, this is a sign of "bad" bacterial overgrowth and a sure sign of the presence of endotoxin. In fact, it's one of the main reasons many people feel better on a ketogenic low-carb diet or carnivore (all meat) diet—by the nature of these diets, they have eliminated the starchy carbs and fiber that were feeding the bacteria and increasing the endotoxin.

If, after three days, you feel better, now you can start adding food back into the diet. Start by adding a food that you would like to eat from the high-insoluble fiber list we've put together (shown below) and notice if you have any reactions over the next few days. Add only one new food every few days, so that, if you have any negative reaction, you will know which food caused it. Many people will notice that after adding a certain food back in, they don't feel as well as they had been feeling.

Here is a list of high-insoluble fiber foods:
- beans
- lentils
- dried apricots, figs, and prunes
- blueberries
- pears
- plums
- strawberries
- broccoli
- brussel sprouts
- carrots
- turnips
- beets
- green beans
- kale
- spinach
- collard greens
- potatoes
- squash
- sweet potato
- zucchini
- quinoa
- almonds
- sesame seeds

Keep a daily food diary of all the foods you eat and how you feel throughout the day, making a note of how well you sleep at night and what your energy is like throughout the day. It amazes people when they find out how many different foods they have been eating that have been producing a negative effect on their life, and they never realized it. They certainly would never have attributed it to a particular food. People will report, "I can't believe I used to feel like this all the time" once they start feeling better. Most of us get used to feeling a certain way that may not be great, but it becomes the norm, and we just think it is the way everyone feels.

What this elimination diet will do once you have taken out the foods that create inflammation, endotoxin, and/or food intolerances, is significantly reduce the stress response/cortisol that the body was producing when it was reacting to the inflammatory food/trigger. And when the inflammatory/stress response decreases, this is when you will be able to notice a significant change when you eat something that doesn't agree with you. Many people who are suffering from a number of GI symptoms are taking daily antihistamines like Benadryl or anti-inflammatories like Advil, which decrease their inflammatory symptoms, never thinking that a certain food might actually be causing these problems. People often continue the cycle of negative food reaction, followed by taking an anti-inflammatory or antihistamine medication, and this becomes a never-ending loop.

One symptom that we often see related to food intolerance is people who are "stuffy" all the time and are unable to breathe without taking some type of sinus medication. They just chalk it up to allergies, when really their "stuffiness" is inflammation of their sinuses coming from a histamine response from the food they are eating. Dairy is probably the most common culprit—not just from lactose intolerance. Many brands of milk, even the organic kinds, have added emulsifiers, and cheeses have added enzymes that create histamine and inflammation. Another common symptom of a food intolerance is snoring and sleep apnea. Many spouses tell us about how their partner snored and/or had sleep apnea due to severe congestion until they changed their diet. Once they eliminated the reactive food, they could sleep without ear plugs.

People say that fermented foods are helpful in losing weight and establishing the proper microbiome. This idea has been somewhat controversial. It is also known that fermented foods can increase endotoxin by providing food for any of the bad bacteria that may be living in the GI tract.

Another common culprit for causing significant GI and systemic symptoms can be mold. Many fermented foods contain mold, and, frequently, people have allergic reactions to mold. These symptoms can resemble the symptoms of bacterial overgrowth and endotoxin. The more common symptoms are headaches, sinus troubles, dizziness, and joint pain. Some of the moldy/fermented foods behind these symptoms are the following:

- all types of cheese, but especially hard cheeses, like cheddar, blue cheese, gorgonzola, Swiss, Colby, and parmesan
- vinegar and foods preserved in vinegar, such as salad dressings, mustard, olives, and pickles
- sour cream, buttermilk, and yogurt
- sauerkraut and other fermented vegetables
- canned tomatoes
- alcoholic beverages, primarily beer and wine
- sourdough bread
- preserved meats, like smoked meats, smoked fish, sausages, ham, and bacon
- dried fruits, like mango, raisins, apricots, cranberries, figs, and prunes
- canned juice

After you have determined which foods are causing a problem, such as soluble fiber, resistant/non-resistant starch, or mold, what do you do to heal? It can take weeks to months to heal the GI tract. A good rule of thumb is to give the GI tract at least three months to begin to show signs of improving health: decreased bloating, decreased indigestion, less gas, more regular bowel habits, decreased fatigue, decreased joint pain, improved mood, better-quality sleep, and decreased nasal congestion.

Continue eliminating all the problem foods from the diet as your GI tract heals. That will be an important part of the healing process. This part of the plan is meant to reduce anything that is causing inflammation. The most common gut-inflammatory foods are PUFA, gluten, preservatives, and gums like xanthum, guar, and carrageenan. If you have been following the Phase One part of our eating plan and eliminating PUFA up to this point, you should be well on your way to healing any GI inflammation.

Next, add more insoluble fiber to help move the bowels. Insoluble fiber also acts like a broom in sweeping/eliminating the bacteria from the colon. The longer food remains in the colon, the more the bacteria and endotoxin can migrate to the rest of the body. One of the best things to add to the healthy diet is a shredded carrot salad once daily. We have included this easy recipe for carrot salad that incorporates shredded carrots, coconut oil, and sea salt. You can also add apple cider vinegar to the recipe if you like. Coconut oil is a saturated fat and has antibacterial properties much like an antibiotic. If you eat coconut oil without the carrot to act as a carrier, it will be absorbed quickly in the small intestine without ever making it to the large intestine. When coconut oil is added to the shredded carrot, the raw carrot, being fibrous, acts like a transport carrier and allows it to travel to the large intestine without being digested. Once it reaches the large intestine, it has an antibacterial effect, along with the broom-like action of the insoluble fiber in the carrot.

Here is the recipe:
- 1 cup of shredded carrots
- 1 tbsp coconut oil
- pinch of sea salt
- 1 tsp to 1 tbsp of apple cider vinegar (optional)

Bamboo shoots are another great source of insoluble fiber to add to the diet daily, creating similar effects to the carrot salad.

There are other ways to reduce bacterial overgrowth and endotoxin, through activated charcoal, oregano oil, and extra saturated fats.

One way to reduce bacterial overgrowth and endotoxin is to add activated charcoal with coconut oil no more than twice a week for as long as symptoms persist. Take one teaspoon of charcoal and mix with one teaspoon of coconut oil. The charcoal has the ability to absorb toxins; it also acts as a transport carrier for the oil to carry it to the large intestine to have the antibacterial effect, much like the carrot salad. If you're taking prescription medication, you'll need to check with your healthcare provider before taking the activated charcoal, as it can bind with certain medications and inactivate them.

A common supplement that has an exceptionally good effect on fighting bacterial overgrowth is oregano oil. This has been used by traditional cultures as an antibiotic and antiparasitic herb. Dosing will depend on the strength of the oregano oil; you can generally get good results by following the instructions on the label

Adding extra saturated fat to the diet, like butter, coconut oil, and animal fat has a healing effect on the colon and an anti-inflammatory effect.

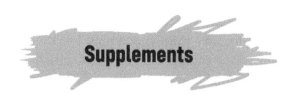

# Supplements

In this section, we will discuss supplements. We will talk not only about nutritional deficiencies and how to prevent them, but also about ways in which we can use some nutritional supplements to get a pharmaceutical-like action, allowing for dramatic effects in changing our physiology and health.

Many healthcare providers will say that, if you eat a healthy diet, there is no need to take nutritional supplements. This would be true in a perfect world where we are eating unprocessed foods that are not grown in mineral-deficient soil. Also, when a person has a long-term deficiency, they may need more supplements than they would normally get in their food. Modern farming results in eating food grown in soil that is deficient in minerals. Our food is now being processed to remove the micronutrients so as to increase the food's shelf life. A good example of this is commercial flour products that have had the bran and germ removed. This depletes vitamin E and all the B vitamins, only to be "fortified" with a few B vitamins and iron. Even the healthiest of diets in the modern world probably could use some help with some types of nutritional supplementation.[1]

We'll look now at some of the major minerals and vitamins that most of us need to supplement.

## Vitamins

Vitamins are actually essential nutrients and can be divided into two main groups: *water-soluble* and *fat-soluble*. Water-soluble vitamins mix in water, whereas fat-soluble vitamins dissolve in fat and are found in fat-containing foods.

Fat-soluble vitamins need fat for absorption. Water-soluble vitamins are not stored in the fat of the body. They are excreted from the body rather than being stored, which means there is less of a chance of build-up and toxicity from consuming too much. Though this is unlikely, some water-soluble vitamins can actually be toxic in high quantities: two examples would be B6 and B12. Since the fat-soluble vitamins are transported and stored in the fat of the body, they have a greater chance to build up and, therefore, a greater chance of becoming toxic over time at higher-than-normal doses.

The government has established a *recommended daily allowance* (RDA) for vitamins, but this rarely considers a person's individual needs and genetics. Many of the RDA recommendations were based on the bare minimum of keeping POWs and prisoners alive during wartimes. Also, for some vitamins and minerals, there is an established upper limit on how much you should ingest. Some people may need more than the RDA, depending on their activity level, overall health level, health conditions, and genetics, which can create the need for one or more particular vitamins or minerals. As we have already discussed, one of the most common causes of inflammation (and one of the most common health problems) in the US is inflammation of the GI tract. This can inhibit the absorption of many nutrients. There are many other health conditions and diseases that result from vitamin and mineral deficiencies. Also, there are subclinical conditions, where the nutrient levels are low, but not low enough to cause the full clinical manifestation(s) of deficiency. However, these subclinical conditions can cause significant health problems.

One of the first vitamin deficiency diseases was discovered in the early 1900s. This condition affected Asian cultures that ate a predominance of white rice in their diet. Due to the removal of bran from brown rice to accommodate the demand, the white rice was stripped of many of its nutrients and, in effect, was then mainly starch. This starch with all the nutrients removed became a mainstay of their diet. The disease was named *beriberi* by the doctor who discovered the condition. This condition causes heart and nervous system failure. Beriberi is caused from a B1 (*thiamine*) deficiency. Health officials say this deficiency is rare in our present times, but is it really? Many researchers believe vitamin B1 deficiencies are common. Could this explain why we have such high occurrence of cardiovascular disease in our American population?

Below, we will list some of the key nutrients and the effects they have on the body and how we can supplement to make sure that our body is operating at its peak efficiency. These are not the only vitamins and minerals the body needs, but we will just focus on the ones that can make the biggest change in optimizing our health.

## The B Vitamins: The Energy Vitamins

The B vitamins are a collection of eight different vitamins. Each one has a different role and function in the body. Since B vitamins are considered water soluble, they do not accumulate in the body like fat-soluble vitamins. This means that we need to consume them on a daily basis. As a whole, the B vitamins control cellular energy, primarily dealing with the conversion of proteins, carbohydrates, and fats into energy. B vitamins affect the energy of each cell and the energy of the whole body. Symptoms of deficiency can include poor muscle tone, drowsiness after eating, heart symptoms like cardiomyopathy, CHF, edema, and neurological symptoms like dementia, neuropathy, numbness, and tingling.

You may hear from the medical establishment that B vitamin deficiencies are rare, but we have found that many people are experiencing subclinical deficiencies that are going untreated. Many people that had some combination of the above symptoms were being treated with prescription medications, but when the B vitamins were supplemented, they reported "miracles" and found that many of their symptoms improved significantly.

The primary sources of the B vitamins are meat, eggs, and whole grains. So, how can a person become B-vitamin deficient when these foods are so abundant? The answer lies in the modern processing of our grain.

As we noted above, this removes the B vitamins, leaving just the starchy part of the plant for us to eat, stripped of many of its nutrients. Changes to the way we process our grain were made in the early 1900s in order to increase the shelf life of baked goods. Have you ever wondered why you do not find bugs in bags of white flour (except weevils that just go to hatch)? Since most or all of the nutrition has been removed, bugs and animals will not eat white flour. They may be smarter than us humans. If you want to try an experiment, put a cup of white flour on your patio and notice that no animals or bugs eat it.

We spoke of the first B vitamin discovered, thiamine (B1), and how with a diet of hulled white rice, people developed beriberi. The beriberi causes heart conditions and is cured just by giving the people a B1 supplement. In 1941, the health of American GIs was a concern, because they had these nutritional deficiencies. The FDA realized that the nutrition was being stripped out of the processed wheat; they mandated that it be "fortified" with thiamine (B1), riboflavin (B2), niacin (B3), and iron. The problem now, however, is that these are many more vitamins that are missing from processed foods. Secondly, many people are eating fewer flour products, so this can lead to subclinical deficiencies. Another common cause of B vitamin deficiency is when many people either decrease or eliminate animal products from their diet. Animal products such as meat, eggs, and fish are high in B vitamins.

Just because you're incorporating foods into your diet with B vitamins doesn't mean your body is processing them. One way to determine how many vitamins you're consuming and the amount of the B vitamins you need is by using an online tool, like an online cronometer.

We recommend that everyone should calculate their B vitamin intake, or—just to be safe—supplement with either individual B vitamins or a B complex. There are a few of the B vitamins that we want to look at that may be supplemented in higher than RDA doses to get the best physiological effect. This means that we can actually change the physiology of the body with supplementation.

Below are a few of the B vitamins that give great results through supplementation if/when a person is either clinically or subclinically deficient.

## B1, Thiamine

We just spoke about thiamine deficiency causing beriberi. B1 deficiency is called the "great imitator of diseases" because it can mimic similar symptoms to many diseases and conditions. Since it plays such a major role in the energy production and carbohydrate metabolism of the body, the most common symptom is fatigue. But it can cause many more symptoms; below are just some of the more common symptoms:

- fatigue
- irritability
- depression
- anxiety
- brain fog
- high blood sugar
- loss of appetite
- stomach fullness
- muscle weakness
- blurred vision
- tingling sensation of the extremities
- insomnia
- enlarged heart
- increased pulse rate
- sleep apnea
- vertigo
- exercise intolerance

As you can see, these are many of the symptoms that are common in our society today. Possibly the most common symptom people are experiencing today is fatigue. Is it just fatigue or a deficiency of thiamine? One of the most important benefits for people trying to lose weight is to supplement generously with vitamin B1, thiamine. Without enough thiamine, we will be unable to metabolize carbs. The body uses twice as much thiamine to burn carbs as it does fat. These symptoms can resolve with adequate intake of B1. Many people feel an immediate effect from their first dose of B1, but, for others, it may take a few months of supplementing to feel its full effects. Thiamine has no known toxicity! The RDA for men is 1.2 milligrams per day; for women over eighteen years, 1.1 mg/day; however, this is often not adequate for optimal health.

The most common form of B1 supplement is thiamine hydrochloride. This is usually adequate for most people, but some people respond better to another form that is fat soluble and may work better at replenishing any thiamine deficiency. This fat-soluble form of B1 is allithiamine, which is a component found in garlic and which was discovered in the 1950s. Another type of fat-soluble B1 discovered by Japanese researchers is *benfotiamine*. For supplementation, use 50–100 mg/day thiamine hydrochloride or 50 mg/day of either allithiamine or benfotiamine. The best food sources for B1 are potatoes, liver, eggs, pork, and coffee.

## B2, Riboflavin

Next, we want to look at B2, riboflavin. The symptoms of riboflavin deficiency may include skin conditions, swelling of the mouth, cracks at the corners of the mouth, cracked lips, thinning hair, fertility issues, sore throat, itchy and red eyes, and liver and nervous system dysfunction.

The RDA for B2, riboflavin is 1.3 mg/day for men and 1.1 for women. Some experts say our true needs are probably closer to 2–5 mg/day. The best food sources for B2, riboflavin are liver, cheese, eggs, and kidneys. Riboflavin/vitamin B2 can be taken as an oral supplement, individually, or in topical form as a B-complex combination liquid vitamin supplement.

## B3, Niacin

Like the rest of the B vitamins, niacin plays a big role in converting proteins, carbs, and fats into energy. Niacin has also been used successfully to lower cholesterol. Niacin is one form of B3 that causes red flushing of the skin. B3 can be toxic to the liver if consumed in large doses. Another form of B3 is *niacinamide* (*nicotinamide*) and one that we can use to get dramatic health effects. Of note, niacinamide does not cause flushing or liver damage.

Symptoms of niacin deficiency include the following:
- fatigue
- poor memory
- depression
- headaches
- skin problems

In fact, a common symptom is cracks in the heels of the feet, which many women have scraped off without thinking about it when they have their pedicures. Niacinamide is converted into its most active form—*nicotinamide adenine dinucleotide* (NAD). Not to get overly technical, but NAD is a major component of energy production in the form of ATP inside the cell (as part of the process, it then gains a hydrogen atom and becomes NADH). Recent research has shown one of the best predictors of health is to have a high NAD to NADH ratio. There are many diseases, including age-associated metabolic disorders—such as diabetes and cancer, neurodegenerative diseases, and mental disorders—that are associated with lowered NAD levels. When there is decreased NAD, there will be mitochondrial dysfunction and increased aging. In fact, just aging alone can cause a decrease in NAD. Research has shown that increasing NAD can have significant anti-aging properties.[2]

Supplementation with NAD+ precursors have beneficial effects on body weight, energy metabolism, mitochondrial function, insulin sensitivity, glucose tolerance, oxidative stress response, fatty liver, weight gain, and Alzheimer's. At this time in the COVID-19 pandemic, there are now studies that show the coronavirus disrupting NAD+ production and utilization. Niacin supplementation has been found to aid in limiting the destructive effects of the virus, and supplementing may be beneficial in speeding the time to recovery. This is understandable since most health conditions interfere with energy production of the cell.[3]

Taking niacinamide shows a wide range of positive health benefits without any negative effects. We recommend starting with 100 mg niacinamide once per day. It is best to take with carbohydrates; due to its role in converting carbs into energy, it can cause a drop in blood sugar. The best food sources for niacin are beef and fish.

## B6, Pyridoxine

B6, pyridoxine, plays a major role in mood because it is needed to create neurotransmitters, such as dopamine, the feel-good neurotransmitter. Vitamin B6, pyridoxine, can also convert amino acids into glucose when you have low blood sugar. It helps your body convert *ammonia*—a byproduct of protein metabolism—into urea, which is then excreted in the urine. B6 helps eliminate *homocysteine*, which is an amino acid that in high levels has been linked to heart disease. Vitamin B6, pyridoxine, also helps eliminate the body's allergic histamine response.

Common symptoms from a B6 deficiency are:

- irritability
- depression
- confusion
- anxiety
- insomnia
- skin problems (similar to a B2 deficiency)
- anemia
- hypoglycemia (low blood sugar)

Though B6, pyridoxine, is a water-soluble vitamin, unlike B1 and B2, you can get too much of it if taken in high doses. The RDA for B6 is 1.3 mg/day for most adults. To avoid toxicity, we recommend starting with low doses around 10 mg/day and working up slowly to a maximum of 100 mg/day. B6 toxicity symptoms usually go away as soon as you stop supplementing. Food sources for B6 are chicken, eggs, liver, meat, carrots, and bananas.

There are other B vitamins: B5 (pantothenic acid), B7 (biotin), B9 (folate), and B12 (cobalamin), all of which play important roles in energy production and health but don't necessarily benefit from higher than physiological doses.

One exception might be vitamin B12 regarding a vegan diet. A vegan diet restricts all animal products like dairy, meat, eggs, and cheese. B12 is found only in animal food products, so those adhering to a vegan diet will become vitamin-B12 deficient unless they take a daily or weekly supplement containing B12.

To make sure you are getting enough of each of the B vitamins, we recommend that you increase the quantity of high-B vitamin-containing foods—i.e., animal products like meat, eggs, and fish, or more whole unprocessed grains. The other way is to supplement daily, either individually or with a combination B-complex vitamin. The main issue with a B complex supplement is that the dosage of vitamin

B6 is usually higher than necessary and may increase the possibility of levels becoming toxic.

## The Fat-Soluble Vitamins

Fat-soluble vitamins dissolve in fat and, therefore, are more readily stored in fat tissue and in the liver. This means that if taken in high quantities, fat-soluble vitamins can become toxic since they are not excreted out of the body in the urine like water-soluble vitamins.

We can generally see significant health benefits and optimization when we replace deficiencies in the fat-soluble vitamins because they play a major role in immune system function and in the production and regulation of hormones. The four major fat-soluble vitamins are vitamin A, vitamin D, vitamin E, and vitamin K.

## Vitamin A, Retinol

Vitamin A is found in animal products like beef, chicken, fish, dairy, and, especially, liver. This is considered the source of the pre-formed vitamin that would include retinol, retinal, and retinoic acid. It is the usable form of vitamin A in the small intestine. Another form is the provitamin A, meaning it must be converted into its usable form; these include carotenoids like beta-carotene, and these are generally found in plant foods.

Let's look at all the important things vitamin A does. It controls growth and differentiation of all the cells in the body, as well as gene expression. It is needed for eye health and vision. Vitamin A deficiency is the leading cause of preventable blindness in the world. It plays a major role in the normal functioning of the immune system, so much so that it has been called "the anti-infection vitamin." In fact, vitamin A deficiency is considered a nutritionally acquired, immunodeficiency disease. Vitamin A also plays a major role in the production of the master thyroid hormone.[4] If deficient in vitamin A, synthesis of thyroid hormones is significantly decreased.

Vitamin A has been used to treat skin conditions such as acne and psoriasis. The drug Accutane, used to treat cystic acne, is a synthetic retinoid.[5] Vitamin A has also shown promise in reducing cancers of the skin, breast, colon, prostate, and liver.[6]

One of the reasons for many of the benefits of vitamin A is due to its ability to balance out effects of estrogen dominance.[7] Vitamin A decreases cortisol, and, by doing this, it can help to decrease the body's stress response.[8] Another great anti-inflammatory benefit of vitamin A is its anti-endotoxin effect. It has been shown to suppress toll-like receptors (TLRs) that are responsible for many different inflammatory by-products.[9]

One of the most common warnings about supplementing with Vitamin A, as with the other fat-soluble vitamins, is the chance for significant toxicity. This tends to be extremely overstated. In some studies, the dosage used was 300,000–500,000 IU/day for months, with only limited toxicity to skin and mucous membranes.[10] But, even at these substantial doses, studies did not show any liver toxicity, which is the typical stated concern when it comes to vitamin A supplementation.

The RDA for vitamin A is 3,000 IU/day. The most common food sources for vitamin A are liver, eggs, and full-fat dairy. A more helpful dosage of vitamin A is 10,000 IU/day in retinol palmitate or retinal acetate forms. This provides enhanced immune response, healthy skin, and proper thyroid function.

## Vitamin D

Vitamin D may be the most important supplement we can take nowadays. Vitamin D as a vitamin is actually a misnomer. It really is not a vitamin at all; it is a steroid hormone. It is often called the "sunshine vitamin" because it is made when sunlight reacts with cholesterol in the skin. The vitamin D produced is then carried to the liver and kidneys to convert it to its active form.

One of the main functions of vitamin D is to increase absorption of calcium from the intestines into the bloodstream. Vitamin D plays an important role in the mineralization of bone formation. This can be seen in young people that are deficient in vitamin D. They will develop bone deformities of the legs, a condition more commonly known as "rickets." In older adults, a vitamin D deficiency can lead to osteoporosis.

Possibly more important than bone health is the positive benefits vitamin D has on the immune system.[11] Research consistently shows that a deficiency of vitamin D influences increased autoimmune conditions and increased susceptibility to infections. In fact, Dr. Anthony Fauci, the lead scientist of the COVID-19 task force and director of the NIH, has recommended taking vitamin D to help in the possible prevention of COVID-19. Per Dr. Fauci, "If you're deficient in vitamin D, that does have an impact on your susceptibility to infection. I would not mind recommending, and I do it myself, taking vitamin D supplements."[12]

In another 2020 study on COVID-19, results showed that vitamin D reduced risks of COVID-19 by decreasing risk of infection, severe cases, hospitalization, ICU care, and risk of death from the virus. The study recommended dosage of 10,000 IU/day and that elderly should probably double that amount to 20,000 IU/day. The increased dosage for the elderly was due to their lowered rate of absorption of vitamin D.[13]

However, the most compelling reason to get enough vitamin D levels is its positive effects in protection against various forms of cancer.[14] Cancer is currently the second leading cause of death in the US. Higher levels of vitamin D were found to be protective against breast cancer and colorectal cancer. In addition, higher levels of vitamin D have shown benefits in protecting against diabetes and depression.

The RDA of vitamin D is currently a pitiful 800 IU per day for adults. A more effective dose would be somewhere in the range of 5,000–10,000 IU/day of vitamin D3 for anyone who is not getting full-body exposure to sunlight. This is especially important for darker-skinned people. The reason for increased supplementation is that darker skin is much less efficient at converting cholesterol to active vitamin D. A lighter-skinned person may make 10,000 IU of active vitamin D3 within twenty to thirty minutes of full body exposure, whereas it may take hours for a darker-skinned person to make the same amount.

Although vitamin D is a fat-soluble vitamin, doses of 10,000 IU/day have not appeared to create any significant complications of toxicity. In fact, one study from 2017 reported that there was an error in calculation of the RDA for vitamin D, suggesting that a more appropriate RDA would be 8,895 IU/day for adults.[15]

## Vitamin E, Tocopherols/Tocotrienols

Vitamin E is a great vitamin with many health benefits. Vitamin E is at the top of the list for making sure that we have adequate supplementation. As a fat-soluble vitamin, it exists in eight different forms. The form *alpha-tocopherol* is the form that most top-selling supplements contain, but supplements with mixed tocopherols have better overall effects. Vitamin E is considered a major antioxidant, meaning it protects cells from free radical damage.[16] Though this is important, it is far more than just an antioxidant.

Once known as the "fertility" vitamin, vitamin E increases fertility in both women and men. One of the ways it increases fertility is by opposing the effects of estrogen.[17] The effect of high estrogen includes clot formation and fibrosis, both of which have a detrimental effect on fertility. Doctors have used vitamin E with great success in treating all kinds of circulatory diseases, such as blood clots, hypertension, heart disease, and diabetes.[18] Vitamin E deficiency can lead to atrophy of testicles, brain, and/or muscles. Also, vitamin E can have a great effect on nerves. When animals were fed a vitamin E-free and vitamin C-free diet, they became paralyzed.

For men, one of the greatest benefits of vitamin E may be the increase of testosterone, due to vitamin E being an aromatase inhibitor.[19] As we covered earlier in the book, aromatase is the enzyme that converts testosterone into estrogen, causing low testosterone levels in both men and women.

One of the biggest effects of vitamin E is the way it protects the body from PUFA. In previous chapters, we discussed how toxic PUFA is on the body. Vitamin E causes direct degradation of the polyunsaturated fats before they can do damage to the cells.[20] It also protects and improves the energy production of the mitochondria.[21] Vitamin E can be found in foods such as wheat germ, nuts, seeds, green leafy vegetables, and avocados.

The RDA of vitamin E is 15 mg/day. The US National Health and Nutrition Examination Survey III (NHANES III) conducted a survey between 2003 and 2006, looking at daily intake of vitamin E with a sample population of 18,063 people. They found that 93% of American adults were under the recommended daily requirement of 15 mg/day.[22] A more beneficial dose for vitamin E is 100 IU/day.

You will find studies and some sources recommending higher doses, but the risk/benefit ratio for the higher dosing regimens is at times problematic.

## Vitamin K

There are many forms of vitamin K, but we will focus on just two. Although they have different functions in the body, the two most important types of vitamin K are K1 (phylloquinone) and K2 (menaquinone). The main benefit of vitamin K1 is blood clotting and preventing excessive bleeding. K1 is mostly found in green leafy vegetables.

The form of vitamin K that has the biggest and most dramatic effect on health is K2. Food sources of K2 are meats, egg yolks, and cheeses.[23] Vitamin K2 has a balancing effect with vitamin D. Vitamin D helps the absorption of calcium from the GI tract into the bloodstream, and K2 moves the calcium from the blood into the bone. Without K2, the calcium won't be able to enter the bone and will likely enter the tissues, causing calcification of soft tissue and arteries.[24] K2 has been shown to lower arterial calcification which, in turn, should lower risk of cardiovascular disease.[25] K2 also inhibits prostaglandins, which play a key role in the inflammatory process. Some studies show that K2 is an aromatase inhibitor, like vitamin E, which means it can also increase testosterone levels through the inhibition of estrogen.[26]

The best type of K2 to supplement with is K2 (MK-4). There is no known toxicity with this K2 form of vitamin K, even though vitamin K is considered a fat-soluble vitamin. We recommend taking 1 mg/day with 800–1,400 mg/day of calcium to insure increased bone density. The recommended RDA for vitamin K currently is typically 90–1,200 mcg/day for adults, but these recommendations do not differentiate between the different forms of K2.

## Minerals

Now that we have covered the main vitamins that we need to supplement, we need to talk about minerals. It is said that we go mineral deficient before we go vitamin deficient. Minerals are inorganic materials that the body requires for many essential functions. In fact, they are needed for almost all functions of the body. Some minerals are needed in larger amounts, and there are some minerals that are needed in only small amounts; these are called trace minerals.

Some of the minerals that are needed in larger quantities are calcium, magnesium, phosphorus, sodium, chloride, and potassium. The trace minerals we need include iron, selenium, zinc, copper, iodine, boron, and fluoride. Even though we need smaller amounts of trace minerals, that does not mean they are less important. Most people don't really need to supplement iron and/or fluoride because we tend to get sufficient quantities of these trace minerals in our daily diet.

We could fill an entire book on the need for and the effects of minerals, but we will just highlight some of the more important functions and which ones we need to supplement. Two main reasons we become mineral deficient is the lack of minerals in the soil due to over-farming, causing the vegetables to contain fewer minerals, as well as the lack of well and spring water that contain minerals.

Let's start with the most abundant minerals in the body.

## Calcium

Calcium is recognized as the most abundant mineral in the body; however, most people are still in need of supplementing due to a fairly limited amount obtained through our diets. Most people have heard about calcium and the need for it to build strong bone and dental health, but that is just one function of many for this important and essential mineral. Calcium plays an important role in intracellular signaling for the body's metabolic processes. It is needed for the transmission of nerve impulses, and it also controls muscle contraction, including the involuntary contractions that pump blood through the heart. In addition, calcium plays a role in optimizing blood pressure and the body's ability to stop and control bleeding. Another important benefit of calcium is that it regulates energy production in the process of glycolysis and the Krebs cycle.[27]

One of the most important benefits of calcium may be the positive effect it has on the immune system. Calcium molecules will actually surround foreign matter, which then identifies this foreign matter for *phagocytes*. Phagocytes are important players in the immune system because they act like little "Pac-Men" and gobble up foreign invaders. The actions of these phagocytes are inhibited with low blood calcium levels.[28]

Calcium has also been shown to play an important role in fighting infections, as illustrated in a 1998 study performed at Linköping University in Sweden. This study shows that the body's ability to kill the tuberculosis bacteria was inhibited when the cell's calcium levels were low, and its ability to kill the tuberculosis bacteria was enhanced when there was a sufficient amount of calcium in the body.

In addition, calcium is known to protect the GI tract against infections from E. coli and can relieve symptoms of diarrhea and help with weight loss as well.[29] It has also been shown in multiple studies that critically ill patients in hospitals often have low levels of calcium, which has been shown to correlate with the severity of the illness.[30]

Here are some of the symptoms of calcium deficiency:
- tachycardia (increased pulse)
- cramps—muscular and intestinal/GI
- fever
- nosebleeds
- bleeding gums
- coughing
- insomnia
- osteoporosis
- hyperirritability
- low blood pressure

The best foods for calcium are dairy, green leafy vegetables, and sesame seeds/almonds. We recommend getting at least 800–1,400 mg/day. The most common forms of calcium supplements are calcium carbonate, calcium citrate, and/or calcium lactate. It doesn't matter much which one of these forms of calcium you choose, although some may debate the advantage of one over another. Our preferred calcium supplement is calcium carbonate in powder form added to juice.[31] It is important, however, to make sure you are getting enough vitamin D to be able to absorb the calcium that you consume. (See vitamin D section above for recommended amounts.)

## Magnesium

Magnesium is the second most abundant mineral in the body. It is used by over three hundred enzymatic reactions in the body. Though we usually think of calcium as the mineral for bone health, magnesium plays a vital role in bone health as well.[32] There have been several studies that show that a higher daily intake of magnesium can decrease osteoporosis in post-menopausal women.[33]

Magnesium also plays a role in muscle contraction and relaxation, an opposing effect to calcium.

Here are some of the other benefits of magnesium:
- lowers blood pressure
- improves blood sugar/diabetes
- decreases C-Reactive Protein and inflammation
- helps prevent migraines
- fights depression/anxiety
- may boost athletic performance
- improves PMS symptoms
- needed for energy production
- involved in DNA repair

Here are some symptoms of magnesium deficiency:
- fatigue
- muscle weakness
- irregular heartbeat
- muscle twitches
- cramps
- depression/anxiety
- osteoporosis
- asthma

Some predictions are that 50–75% of the US population is magnesium deficient.[34] Foods that are high in magnesium are dark chocolate, avocado, almonds, cashews, black beans, pumpkin seeds, quinoa, halibut, salmon, and Swiss chard, as noted below.

| Food | Magnesium Content | Serving size |
|---|---|---|
| Dark chocolate | 64 mg | 1 oz |
| Avocado | 58 mg | 1 medium size |
| Nuts | 82 mg | 1 oz |
| Beans | 120 mg | 1 cup |
| Pumpkin seeds | 150 mg | 1 oz |
| Whole grains | 65 mg | 1 oz |
| Fatty fish (halibut, salmon) | 178 mg | 1/2 fillet |
| Banana | 37 mg | 1 large |
| Leafy greens | 157 mg | 1 cup |

The RDA for magnesium is 420 mg/day for men and 320 mg/day for women. We recommend that a person supplement with 400–600 mg/day. The most common forms of magnesium supplements are magnesium citrate, magnesium glycinate, and magnesium malate. One of the common side effects, and often intended effects, of higher doses of magnesium is loose bowels (commonly used for bowel prep prior to a colonoscopy). Magnesium malate tends to be better tolerated, as it does not have this effect on the GI tract.

## Sodium

Sodium is essential for life and health. It is in our diet usually in the form of table salt. Table salt is *sodium chloride*, which means it is approximately half sodium and half chloride. Another type of salt not often used in the diet is *sodium bicarbonate*, which is baking soda—half sodium and half bicarbonate.

Sodium may be one of the most controversial and maligned minerals of them all, which stems from the belief that salt causes high blood pressure and swelling. This became the mantra of the medical community when diuretics were first introduced in the mid-1900s—a marketing move to make the diuretics more attractive. In a small percentage of people, sodium may cause increased blood pressure and/or swelling, but, for most people, this is not the case.[35] Actually, sodium, along with albumin, is necessary for maintaining blood volume. With low sodium, the albumin in the bloodstream is unable to prevent water from leaving and seeping into the tissues of the body. So, as the blood volume becomes lower, the tissues become swollen.

One side effect of low salt levels is that the adrenal glands produce a hormone called aldosterone, which actually allows your kidneys to conserve salt. This has a wasting effect on *potassium*, another important mineral that we will discuss in a moment. An increase in aldosterone also causes the adrenals to produce more of the stress hormones adrenaline and cortisol.

There are many studies that show that salt restriction lowers blood pressure a few points, but this does not mean increased health. When a few extra grams of salt were consumed in one study, there was a 36% reduction in coronary events. Studies have also shown an inverse relationship between salt consumption and mortality rates, such that when salt consumption is higher, mortality is lower.[36]

More recently, lowered salt intake has been linked in medical research to the following conditions:

- metabolic syndrome[37]
- insulin resistance[38]
- increased heart disease and mortality
- decreased cognition for older adults

Research from Harvard Medical School showed that when healthy people were placed on a low salt diet of 1/5 of a teaspoon, they developed insulin resistance in just seven days.[39] The recommended dosage from the FDA is 2,300 mg/day of sodium, which is approximately one teaspoon of table salt. The average person consumes 1.5–1.75 teaspoons per day. Although this is higher than the

FDA recommendations, this is approximately half the amount of salt consumed by Americans between the War of 1812 and World War II, which, for that almost one-hundred-year period, was roughly equivalent to 3.3 teaspoons per day. This is to illustrate that even with salt consumption over and above the recommended FDA allowances at the time, metabolic syndrome, insulin resistance, dementia, and cognitive impairment with aging were not as endemic as they are today, with much lower FDA recommended allowances of sodium.

## How Much Salt?

Though there is not a general consensus on the perfect amount of salt at the present time, it appears that 1.5 to 1.75 teaspoons per day is a good starting place. Of course, this is assuming the person does not have kidney or heart disease—in that case, there will be some need to limit salt intake. Himalayan sea salt is a common and acceptable alternative to standard table salt, as is Celtic sea salt.

## Potassium

Potassium an important mineral. Though not discussed much, this may be the most common nutritional deficiency. It is an electrolyte that propagates electrical impulses. Its main function is to help muscles work, including the heart and lungs. Potassium plays a role in the following:

- normal fluid balance
- blood pressure
- nerve impulses
- muscle contraction
- digestion
- heart rhythm

Here are some symptoms of potassium deficiency:
- extreme fatigue
- high blood pressure
- constipation[40]
- muscle weakness

- insomnia
- abnormal heart rhythm
- anxiety
- muscle cramps
- high insulin
- sugar cravings

Here are some of the causes of potassium deficiency:
- diet
- diuretics
- Ketogenic diet
- vomiting
- high cortisol
- excessive water intake
- decreased fruit/vegetable intake

The recommended daily amount of potassium is 4,700 mg/day. When we look at the diet of most people, their diet typically falls significantly short of this amount. To give an example why: most people have heard bananas contain a lot of potassium, which they do. A banana contains around 425 mg of potassium. This would mean that a person would need to eat eleven bananas every day to reach the recommended daily amount of potassium! Since the main sources of potassium come from fruits and vegetables, and most people consume fewer of these due to the abundance of processed foods, it's important to supplement at the higher end of the recommended daily amount in order to maintain adequate potassium levels for optimal health.

Below is a list of foods that contain high potassium:

| Food | Serving Size | Potassium Content (mg) |
|---|---|---|
| Spinach | ½ cup | 420 mg |
| Banana | 1 | 425 mg |
| Potato white (baked) | 1 | 941 mg |
| Sweet potato | 1 | 542 mg |
| Orange juice | 1 cup | 496 mg |

| Plain yogurt, nonfat | 8 ounces | 531 mg |
|---|---|---|
| Salmon, Atlantic, wild | 3 ounces | 534 mg |
| Tuna, yellowfin, cooked | 3 ounces | 448 mg |
| Avocado | ½ cup | 364 mg |
| Apricots, dried, uncooked | ¼ cup | 378 mg |
| Skim milk (nonfat) | 1 cup | 382 mg |
| Kidney beans, cooked | ½ cup | 357 mg |

The best form of potassium supplement is potassium bicarbonate—how much depends on what the person's daily intake is. Most people can benefit from 100–500 mg/day. Caution should be exercised with any type of kidney disease or known cardiac arrhythmia.

## Selenium

Selenium is a mineral that is present in the soil and picked up by plants. This means that how much of the mineral is in the food is largely dependent on how much is in the soil. As we just mentioned, with modern farming, this has become a problem since crops now are continuously grown in the same field, which depletes the soil and thereby depletes the minerals. Selenium is needed for good thyroid health and optimal overall metabolism. A deficiency of selenium has been associated with hypothyroidism and Hashimoto's thyroiditis.

Other benefits of selenium include the following:
- powerful antioxidant
- may reduce risk of cancer
- boosts immune system
- may protect against heart disease
- may prevent mental decline

Foods that are high in selenium are oysters, Brazil nuts, yellowfin tuna, eggs, sardines, sunflower seeds, halibut, shiitake mushrooms, and chicken breast. We recommend tolerable upper limit of selenium at 200 mcg/day. The RDA is currently set at 55 mcg/day.[41]

## Zinc

Zinc is another mineral that is needed for health; it is often paired with selenium. Zinc is used by over one hundred enzymes in the body. One of the most important benefits of zinc is helping to boost the immune system. This is why you see zinc added to lozenges in over-the-counter cold remedies and in popular products like Airborne ©.

Another important benefit of zinc is in preserving and improving prostate health for men and increasing levels of testosterone production. Zinc is important to many functions, as noted below:

- boosting immune function
- protein synthesis
- wound healing
- DNA synthesis
- cell division
- prostate health

Oysters contain the most zinc of any food. Other foods high in zinc are meat, poultry, beans, nuts, whole grains, and dairy products. One difficulty with whole grains is that they contain a substance called phytates that inhibit the absorption of zinc. As a result, there is not much zinc the body can absorb from whole grains.

The recommended tolerable upper limit for zinc is 40 mg/day. Zinc can cause nausea and GI distress, especially on an empty stomach, even at the doses that we are recommending. When taking the zinc with food, these effects are generally minimal. Research shows that zinc prevents entry of the coronavirus into the cells and thereby greatly reduces the severity and the mortality associated with COVID-19.[42]

## Copper

Copper is another trace mineral. It is involved in metabolism, energy production, iron metabolism, connective tissue synthesis, and neurotransmitter synthesis. Copper may also be protective against cardiovascular disease and Alzheimer's disease. Some foods high in copper are shellfish, animal organ meats, whole grains, and any kind of chocolate. The recommended tolerable upper limit for copper intake is 10,000 mcg/day.[43]

## Bone Broth/Collagen/Gelatin/Glycine

When we talk about supplementation, most people would never think that we would include gelatin in this discussion. In reference to gelatin, we're not really talking about Jell-O™ brand gelatin. Gelatin is actually the cooked form of collagen. It is the gelatinous substance that we see on top of chicken soup made with the whole chicken and then cooled.

Gelatin/collagen is found in the bones, skin, and hooves of animals. Traditional cultures have always used the whole animal for food, and we still find many cultures today that continue to utilize the whole animal for its food source. We see this in traditional foods such as ox tail soup, chicken feet soup, fish head soup, traditional chicken matzo ball soup, and what has recently become popular and trendy, bone broth. What all these dishes have in common is that they are cooked to release the gelatin/collagen from the more non-traditional animal parts. It is only recently that the American culture has limited its source of animal meat to the muscle meat.

The difference between muscle meat and gelatin is in the amino acid content. Muscle meat is high in the amino acids *tryptophan* and *cysteine*. Both of these amino acids inhibit thyroid function and interfere with energy production in the mitochondria. Tryptophan is the precursor to serotonin. Serotonin in the body (outside of the brain) causes an increase in cortisol, inflammation, suppresses the immune system, and causes fibrosis of tissue. Gelatin contains little tryptophan. It is high in the amino acids glycine and proline. Glycine acts similar to *GABA*, which is the brain's anti-anxiety neurotransmitter. Most people report significant reduction in anxiety and improvement in sleep when incorporating gelatin into their daily diet.

Reported benefits of taking collagen/gelatin include the following:
- improved joint health
- healthier hair, skin, and nails
- increased muscle mass

- improved gut health
- improved mood
- reduced anxiety
- improved sleep

We recommend adding bone broth, collagen, gelatin, or glycine to the diet daily. Bone broth would be the preference because it is a whole food and has many other important nutrients. Of course, collagen and gelatin have more nutrients than taking only glycine, but if you are unable to get collagen or gelatin, then taking glycine is better than not incorporating collagen/gelatin into the diet at all.

Recommended daily intake of glycine is 1,000–3,000 mg, two times daily.

Though there are many vitamins and minerals we did not discuss, most of them are usually obtained in sufficient quantities through the diet.

---

### Takeaways from Supplements

1. In our day and age, the processing of our food leads most of us to have ongoing nutritional deficiencies.

2. Many of today's RDA recommendations are inaccurate, as they were based on the bare minimum of keeping POWs alive during wartime.

3. Vitamin D may be the most important supplement we can take nowadays. The five supplements that we recommend to everyone are vitamin D3, calcium, magnesium, B-complex and vitamin K2.

---

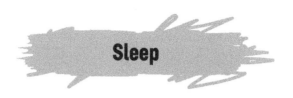
# Sleep

## The Forgotten Performance Enhancer

Sleep is better than any performance-enhancing drug you can take:

- Sleep by itself will not make you healthy, but you can't have health without it.
- Getting the right kind of sleep is the single most effective thing you can do to reset the brain and body each day.
- The World Health Organization has declared sleep loss an epidemic throughout all industrialized nations.

We all sleep every night of our lives (at least, we try), and we have heard that we should get eight hours a night, but why are so few of us getting the recommended amount?

Sleep can be one of our greatest health boosters or one of our greatest health suppressors. It is estimated by the CDC that 35% of Americans get less than seven hours of sleep per night. Forty% of people in the forty-to-fifty-nine age group reported getting less than the recommended eight-hour sleep amount.

All living things sleep—plants, ocean life, mammals, reptiles, birds, and everything in between! Every species has a different amount of sleep that it needs for optimal function. Elephants need 4 hours, gorillas 9.4 hours, squirrels 15.9 hours, and lions and tigers 15 hours. No matter what anyone might tell you, we humans need seven to nine hours, with most of us needing a good, solid eight hours per night for our optimal function. So, in light of this, the true definition of being "sleep deprived" is considered less than seven hours per night.

Humans are the only species that voluntarily sleep deprives itself. How many times do you stay up trying to complete the project for work or cramming for a test the next day? What about binge watching one more episode on Netflix? What happens when we don't get enough sleep?

Lack of sleep does the following:

- increases cortisol
- decreases the immune system
- increases our chances of Alzheimer's disease/dementia
- disrupts blood sugar control, increasing our risk for diabetes
- increases food cravings
- causes weight gain and inability to lose fat
- increases blocked arteries, leading to stroke and heart attacks
- is a symptom found in all major psychiatric conditions, including depression, anxiety, and suicide

Sleep is controlled by an internal twenty-four-hour clock, known as our circadian rhythm. The clock is not exactly twenty-four hours. It turns out to be twenty-four hours and fifteen minutes if kept in darkness; however, when we get exposed to any kind of light during the day, our circadian rhythm will reset to twenty-four hours. This internal clock is controlled by an area in the brain located next to the optic nerve.[1]

Melatonin is known as the "darkness" hormone or the "vampire" hormone. A rise in melatonin begins at sunset and acts as the signal, telling the brain and body that it's dark. One of the myths about melatonin is that it will cause you to sleep, but it actually has little influence on the initiation of sleep.

For this reason, melatonin is not actually the best sleep aid for most people who try to use it for insomnia. Where it has shown its effectiveness is with helping signal jet-lagged people that it is time to sleep, allowing them to adapt their sleep cycle to the time zone they happen to be traveling in.

With modern air travel, feeling "jet-lagged" is a real and stressful event. When traveling to a different time zone, it takes at least one day to reset one hour. This means if you travel to Europe and it's a five-hour difference, it can take up to five days or more to correct your internal clock. Studies have found significant abnormalities in airline pilots and flight attendants who routinely travel long international flights. The parts of their brain that control learning and memory had actually physically atrophied, and their short-term memory was notably impaired.

One major problem in the modern world, where most of us must function in the normal 8:00 a.m. to 5:00 p.m. schedule, is that we may have a circadian rhythm that does not match the traditional schedule. A person's daily rhythm is mainly controlled by genetics. We hear about the morning person who jumps out of bed at the crack of dawn ready to go—they make up about 40% of the population. Then there are the night owls who are just getting started when the morning folks are going to bed—this is about 30% of the population. And then we have the "in- betweens" who make up the remaining 30%—they wake up later and go to bed a couple of hours later than everyone else.

For those of us who are night owls, it is not about having discipline and will power to change into a morning person who naturally bounds out of bed first thing in the morning. For the night owl, when waking up early, their brain will stay in a non-wake state during the early morning hours. Therefore, night owls as a group are more often sleep-deprived since they have to try to conform to the traditional schedule society operates on. This can actually put them at risk for a higher incidence of health issues, such as heart attack and strokes, as well as increased rates of cancer, diabetes, depression, and anxiety.

One of the important things that happens when we don't get enough sleep is something called "sleep pressure," which builds up. Sleep pressure is caused by the chemical *adenosine* building up in the brain. Adenosine jumpstarts the desire to sleep and increases each moment we are awake. This is what causes the urge to sleep for most people after being up for twelve to sixteen hours.

This is where coffee has its biggest effects. It works on the neurotransmitter known as adenosine that is important in promoting sleep. The caffeine in coffee decreases the urge to sleep by blocking the adenosine receptor. As long as there is caffeine in your body, adenosine can build up, but the caffeine will prevent it from promoting sleep. Once the caffeine is gone, then there's the big letdown and the crash.[2] The half-life of caffeine for most people is approximately five hours; this means that half the caffeine is still in your body five hours later. If you have a cup of coffee at 5:00 p.m., then, when it's time to sleep at 10:00 p.m., it's like you just drank half a cup of coffee. As you get your full eight hours of sleep during the night, adenosine is depleted, and your system resets. If you don't get enough sleep, then you carry over the adenosine, and, without caffeine, the sleep pressure remains high, and you will be sleepy. This is why so many people stay chronically tired, feeling the ongoing effects of this continuing sleep pressure.

## What Exactly Happens When We Sleep?

Sleep is divided into two phases: REM sleep and non-REM sleep. There are four stages of sleep. The first three stages make up non-rapid eye movement (NREM), and the fourth stage is rapid eye movement (REM). This cycle repeats through the night anywhere from four to five times.

Stage 1 is the start of the sleep cycle and the transition from the waking state to sleep. This stage usually lasts for about five minutes.

Stage 2 is a deeper sleep than stage one. The body temperature begins to drop and breathing becomes more regular. It's during this phase, we think, that our memories from the day are transferred to longer term storage areas in the brain. We spend about 50% of the time asleep in Stage 2, which lasts anywhere from ten to sixty minutes per cycle.

Stage 3 is the deepest part of sleep. The rates of breathing and blood pressure decrease. The brain waves slow to their slowest level, producing delta waves. Because of this, this stage is often called "delta sleep" or slow wave sleep (SWS). During this stage, which lasts any-where from twenty to forty minutes per cycle, people may sleepwalk.

REM is the last stage in the sleep cycle and is called REM because of the rapid eye movement that occurs, which most people have heard about. This is the stage where we dream. Brain activity becomes much more active. During this stage, the brain produces brain waves very similar to those we have when awake. In REM sleep, the body becomes more relaxed and immobilized. This immobilization keeps us from hurting ourselves while we dream. It is estimated that we spend about 20% of our sleep time in this stage.[3]

We cycle through each stage approximately four to five times per night. An important aspect when we think of the stages is that the length of time we spend in each stage changes throughout the night.

We initially start REM sleep about ninety minutes after we have fallen asleep. The first REM stage may last only for a few minutes, but, with each cycle, it will last longer and can last up to an hour as the night goes on. So, if you go to bed late, you will actually decrease the amount of your NREM sleep or deep sleep, as NREM sleep is predominant in the early part of the night; if you wake up too soon, you decrease the amount of REM sleep (dream sleep) that is predominant in the later part of the night.[4]

NREM and REM sleep have different functions other than dreaming and non-dreaming. As we mentioned, NREM sleep takes memories that are being stored in short-term memory and moves them to long-term memory storage. It also has a weeding-out effect, discarding unnecessary information that was created during the day.[5]

REM sleep, besides dreaming, is responsible for stabilizing and consolidating information, then integrating the memories into our model of the world, which aids in problem solving. It also helps process emotions and deal with difficult experiences. A good way to remember this is "being awake is for learning, and sleeping is for remembering." Studies show being sleep-deprived can lower our learning ability by 40%, so staying up late "cramming" for a test or losing sleep to learn something new for work is actually causing you to not remember what you are trying to learn.

Maybe the best demonstration of how sleep deprivation affects concentration and performance is driving a car with too little sleep. Sleep deprivation, getting less than seven hours of sleep, is responsible for 83,000 car crashes per year. Driving in this condition is termed "drowsy driving." How it affects driving can be translated into all areas of life. It decreases your attention span, slows your reaction time, makes you less coordinated, and decreases your ability to make decisions.[6]

When you are not getting the sleep you need, it's as if you are driving drunk. Studies show that being awake eighteen hours is like having a blood alcohol level of 0.05%, and being awake for twenty-four hours is the same as having a blood alcohol level of 0.10%. Since the level for driving while intoxicated (DWI) is 0.08%, missing a night's sleep is like walking around intoxicated.

An important reason that lack of sleep causes so many auto accidents and lapses in concentration in all aspects of your life is what are called microsleeps. This is when you have sudden, short periods of sleep. Some people will feel their eyelids get heavy and close them, or their head will start to nod, but then they awaken with a jerk. Many times, a person's eyes will not close, and the brain is between being asleep and awake, which can be between one and fifteen seconds. Just imagine driving and your brain shuts off for a few seconds at a time without your realizing it or sitting in an important meeting and missing what is said for fifteen seconds. Microsleeping also gives amnesia-like symptoms, so a person may not even remember what was said or done.[7]

There is no doubt that we all can realize how important sleep is. How do you know if you are sleep deprived?

- Do you get less than seven hours of sleep per night?
- Do you fall asleep within minutes of lying in bed?
- Do you have to use an alarm clock to wake up?
- Do you have to have coffee before noon to function?
- Can you fall back to sleep at 10:00 or 11:00 a.m.?
- Do you have to reread text several times just to comprehend it?

If you answered "yes" to any of these questions, you are probably sleep deprived.

## Now, How Do We Get More and Better Sleep?

First, you must make a conscious choice to make it a priority. Just like scheduling meetings at work or knowing that your workday happens between certain times, you have to schedule your sleep time and wake time, if possible, going to bed and getting up at the same time every night, even on weekends. It is easier to know when you need to go to bed once you decide what time you need to get out of bed, and then count backwards to estimate when you need to schedule your bedtime so that you can get a minimum of seven, maximum of nine hours of sleep per night. One of the biggest disruptors of sleep is not keeping to a schedule. So many people will stay up late on the weekends and then sleep late, and then wind up going to bed late on Sunday night, because they aren't tired, and starting the week off on Monday already sleep deprived.[8] It is better to keep to the same schedule, even during the weekends.

A common myth is that you can make up the sleep you missed during the week by sleeping more on the weekend. Unfortunately, this does not work, and, if this is your pattern, you will more than likely continue to suffer a sleep deficit.

Another major disrupter of sleep is due to the convenience of modern lights. Before electricity, most people would go to bed soon after nightfall because of the limited light. Now nightfall has little meaning. It is not only light, but the type of light. Any type of light, but especially the light from fluorescent bulbs, LED lights, and digital screens—i.e., the "blue light spectrum"—suppresses the release of melatonin, the hormone that tells us it is time to sleep. To help combat the effects of light, consider the following:

- Avoid electronic devices such as televisions, phones, computers, and tablets two to three hours before bedtime.
- Use blue light-blocking filters on digital products or use blue light-blocking filter glasses.
- If watching television before bedtime, keep the living room dim (Don't watch TV in your bedroom!).
- Keep your bedroom dark—use blackout curtains if needed and cover any light that may come from electronic devices.

Studies show that people sleep more soundly and deeply when they have a lower body temperature and the room has a lower temperature. If possible, lower the room temperature to 65–66 degrees and cover up with a blanket. If you get hot at night, you can stick your feet out from under the covers. Taking a warm bath before bed will also help lower your body temperature.

One of the most overlooked sleep disrupters that is rarely talked about in the medical community is that of episodes of *hypoglycemia* (low blood sugar) in the middle of the night. If you think about it, if you eat dinner at 6:00 p.m. and then you wake up at 3:00 a.m., that is a nine-hour period. If there is any type of blood-sugar-regulation problem, but not necessarily diabetes, the blood sugar will drop too low while you are sleeping. Many people who wake up between 1:00 and 4:00 a.m. think they have to get up to use the bathroom, but really, their blood sugar levels have dropped. As you have learned, when that happens, cortisol rises, which then tells your body it is time to get up.

An easy solution for this is to eat a small snack with protein, carbs, and fat before you go to bed, which will keep your blood sugar more stable throughout the night.[9]

---

### Takeaways from Sleep

1. The World Health Organization has declared sleep loss an epidemic throughout all industrialized nations. When you're not getting enough sleep, it's as if you're driving drunk!

2. Sleep can be one of the greatest health boosters or one of the greatest health suppressors. Getting the right kind of sleep at night is the single most effective thing we can do to reset the brain and body each day—we can't have optimal health without it!

3. We may have a circadian rhythm that does not match the traditional 8:00 a.m. to 5:00 p.m. work schedule; our circadian rhythm is mainly controlled by genetics.

---

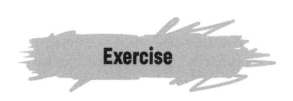

# Exercise

We can consider exercise as the "new superfood." We want to make this a part of our everyday lives. Movement is essential to wellness. You can't really have optimal health and strong bones and joints without moving. The great news is we can accomplish this in a variety of ways. Obviously, strength training and aerobic, high-intensity interval training (HIIT) are important staples that are especially important for weight loss. Walking one hour per day does have good health benefits, but will not necessarily facilitate significant weight loss, so if that's the expectation, don't frustrate yourself; the goal is not to produce cortisol! We can get good results with smaller workout periods over a longer time that will allow us to be more consistent. Expectations, setting small goals to avoid injury, making modifications, and maintaining consistency—these are our goals. If you've been sedentary for some time, like many of us, something as small as walking up one flight of stairs and back down, two different times during a day, can be of big benefit in helping us get started toward our goal of optimal health. And you may already have heard recommendations to park the car a little further from the door, but since a lot of people are working from home now, that may or may not be helpful advice.

These are three types of exercise we want to build into our weekly workout schedule:

- aerobic activity—i.e., low-impact, HIIT (high-intensity interval training), and/or running
- flexibility—i.e., yoga, isometric exercises, or dynamic stretching
- strength training—i.e., weight machines, free weights, calisthenics

With aerobic activity, great benefits can be achieved with small increments of high-intensity interval training. As little as twenty seconds to one minute of activity that raises the heart rate, intermixed with longer sets of active recovery exercise, can go a long way toward helping us transition from the couch or computer screen to a more active and mobile lifestyle. (See "Resources" for list of options.)

Flexibility can be obtained through various yoga poses, isometric exercises, static stretching, or dynamic stretching; the goal is to increase range of motion, lengthen muscles, and avoid injury. Chair exercises (stretching hip flexors) can help alleviate back pain. Being sedentary, as a society, is the new heart-health risk, and sitting, without periods of interrupted activity and movement, can create significant issues with chronic back, neck, and shoulder pain. As many as one in five Americans suffer from chronic pain, and this is not just the elderly. In fact, $80 billion in lost wages occurs each year from missed workdays due to pain among the working population.

Strength training consists of using weight machines, free weights, and calisthenics. This kind of training does not require large amounts of time; for example, doing bicep curls, one set of ten, two different times per day, takes twenty seconds for each set. That is often thought of as "bulking up," or for older women trying to avoid osteoporosis, but actually, building and maintaining muscle is important for all of our bodies as we age.[1] Strength training is essential in protecting us from a certain loss of mobility that can keep us sedentary, which can bring on more inflammation.

Muscles we want to target are the shoulders, back, legs, biceps, triceps, and trunk/core/abdominals. If you're new to strength training and/or exercise, the best way to stay safe is to work with someone on machine-based weights and exercises; in addition, make sure you are confident and knowledgeable about the correct positioning and execution of each of the exercises designed to strengthen your muscles before you workout on your own. Incorrect form or bad execution will most certainly set you up for less-than-optimal results and greatly increase the risk of injury.

There are many other benefits from strength training and/or excercise, some of which are shown below:

- **Helps to increase and maintain muscle mass:** As we age, we lose muscle mass. Strength training can help you maintain and prevent the loss of muscle mass. But how much muscle mass do we actually need? And how do we maintain it once we get it? These are dependent on several factors, one of which is gender. Men typically average 38–54% body weight as muscle mass, whereas women typically average 28–39% of their body weight as muscle mass. This will also depend on age and physical activity levels. For younger adults, typically one set of five to seven exercises with the major muscle groups per week is all that is really needed to maintain their muscle mass; for older adults, however, typically two to three sets of five to seven exercises every four to five days is needed to sustain and maintain adequate muscle mass.

- **Contributes to adequate weight management:** Strength training can and does help to lower body fat by providing more muscle to burn fat at rest.
- **Increases ability to engage in daily activities:** Regular strength training reduces risk of limitations in daily activities due to a lack of adequate muscular fitness. Many daily activities, such as carrying children or groceries, climbing up and down stairs, moving furniture or lifting boxes, taking part in sporting activities or hiking, and even just having to stand for long periods of time, can be factored into our strength training workout.
- **Reduces psychological stress:** Regular exercise is known to reduce the symptoms associated with depression and anxiety; increasing muscle mass will help increase energy and reduce fatigue. Being and feeling stronger has been associated with a more positive self-image.
- **Improves learning and memory:** Exercise increases blood flow to the brain. By doing so, research shows us that just one hour of walking two times per week (that comes out to seventeen minutes a day!) over a six-month period can have lasting effects for learning and memory, increasing the size of our hippocampus—the region in the brain dedicated to new learning and memory.
- **Prevents osteoporosis:** Weight bearing is known to increase bone density.
- **Reduces pain from arthritis:** Maintaining adequate mobility and blood flow to joints limits the incapacitating symptoms and pain often associated with arthritis.

- **Develops a healthier heart:** Regular exercise improves the efficiency of heart function.

Exercise affects our ability to sleep. If we are getting in the habit of regular exercise, doing it in the morning or by early afternoon can raise our internal core temperature. Later on in the evening, the core temperature will fall back to normal, which can induce drowsiness, leading to a deeper sleep. Exercise is also well known to decrease anxiety, and this will also make for better-quality sleep.

Exercise affects stress and inflammation. Exercise is known to increase blood flow to the brain, leading to an increased supply of oxygen-rich blood and other nutrients. This allows the brain to grow in volume, especially in the hippocampal region, which is the area best known for learning and memory. Stress is known to decrease the formation of neurons, which are the brain's basic cells, and this decrease then leads to the development of depression and/or anxiety, especially if the stress is chronic.

Exercise affects the brain. Exercise allows the brain to produce new neurons through a hormone known as *brain-derived neurotrophic factor* (BDNF). Science today tells us that we can build new brain cells at any age. Stress produces increased cortisol levels, which are a marker for inflammation, as you have learned throughout the book. Studies have shown that those with high levels of cortisol in their body lose brain tissue at a faster rate than those with lower cortisol levels.[2] So, exercise is an important tool we have to reverse and counter the effects of chronic stress and inflammation.

## Common Reasons For Not Exercising

The biggest reason given for not exercising is time, or lack of it. We are big proponents of scheduling your workouts, not just leaving them to chance or postponing them on the day's "To Do" list. This is the best way to make sure exercise never happens. Instead, take a few minutes to look at the week ahead and see where and how exercise will be possible. Each day, you can see how you did with your step goal, with staying active, with increasing your mobility, and/or with interrupting sitting or sedentary activities. You can use this information to adjust for the next day's schedule.

The second biggest obstacle to exercising is our perception of what exercise has to be in order to be effective and beneficial. Actually, as mentioned earlier, twenty seconds of weight exercise, thirty seconds of climbing stairs, ten minutes of HIIT workouts, or even thirty minutes of walking briskly each day can add years to your life. So, let's get started!

---

## Takeaways from Exercise

1. We can consider exercise the new "superfood." We want to make this a part of our everyday life.

2. Three types of exercise we want to build into our weekly schedule are aerobic activity, flexibility, and strength training.

3. Movement is essential to wellness. Twenty seconds of weight exercise, thirty seconds of climbing stairs, ten minutes of HIIT workouts, or even thirty minutes of brisk walking each day can add years to your life!

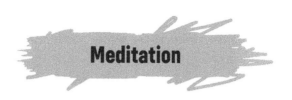

# Meditation

Now we come to the section about meditation. In addition to changing your diet, establishing a regular routine can vastly improve your health and all aspects of your life. Just because we are putting this in now does not mean it should not be a daily priority. Many of you at this moment may just tune out because the word "meditation" can conjure up images of a monk sitting in a funny position in a monastery, or others may think meditation is tied to some religious practice, but actually, this cannot be further from the truth.

Let's first look at what meditation is and what meditation is not. Meditation is silencing the inner chatter of the mind. Most of us have thoughts racing through our mind every waking moment, and we are not even aware much of the time of what we are thinking about. We are usually ruminating over the past, or we are worrying about something in the future that may or may not ever happen; few of us are ever in the present moment, have any periods of silence in our minds, and are able to enjoy what we are experiencing in the moment. Think back to a time when you were at the beach, just watching and listening to the waves, not thinking about anything but being in that moment with the rhythm of the waves; or maybe a time when you were in the mountains watching the sunrise, which felt like the only thing in the world at that moment—that's meditation. So, meditation is really just quieting the mind. In a moment, we will look at some methods on how we can do this.

What meditation is not is some type of religion, or even related to religion. It doesn't require you to believe in any particular god or any god at all. The reason it has been associated with religion is that it has been part of Eastern cultures for thousands of years. For these particular religions, like Buddhism or Hinduism, meditation is a regular part of their spiritual practices. In many forms of Christian religion, daily practices include chanting and/or meditative prayer.

If it helps to get over any preconceived thoughts or images that may come up, whenever we say the word "meditation," we can substitute the word "awareness." When we are practicing awareness, we are able to observe our thoughts—this is the real meaning of meditation.

Before we look at techniques and methods, let's talk about why meditation is an essential part of optimum health and wellness. First, let's look at the benefits of meditation that have been proven scientifically.[1]

Meditation reduces stress, lowering cortisol levels. Since we have discussed throughout this book how bad stress is for you, and that high cortisol levels lead to accelerated aging and systemic inflammation, if this were the only benefit, it would already be well worth the effort. In addition, meditation has been shown to decrease inflammation caused by stress and to improve symptoms of fibromyalgia, irritable bowel disease, and post-traumatic stress disorder.[2]

For these reasons, many of the top companies offer meditation classes and time to meditate at work. Some of the most well-known companies encouraging employees in the practice of daily meditation are Google, Nike, General Mills, Goldman Sachs, and Apple.[3]

Research shows that, when employees meditate, they are less stressed and more productive, and, as a result, the company's health care costs go down. In a 2018 employer-sponsored Health and Wellbeing Survey performed by Fidelity Investments and the National Business Group on Health, results found that 52% of the 163 companies surveyed offered mindfulness, yoga, and/or meditation training.[4]

In fact, studies show that meditation actually changes the brain structure compared to those who do not meditate. People who have been meditating for years show notable increases in the gray matter of the prefrontal cortex. The prefrontal cortex is the area of the brain that is associated with higher levels of thinking, decision-making, and memories. Meditation has also been shown to increase the gray matter in the sensory areas and auditory areas of the brain.[5]

This is great news since one of the effects of aging is that the brain shrinks as we age, and, with meditation, we may be able to prevent this shrinkage from happening or certainly slow the process!

Research has shown that meditation increases the areas of the brain involved in learning, cognition, and emotional control. Meditation can actually shrink the area of the brain that we discussed early in the book, the amygdala, that controls fear and anxiety. Amazingly, these changes can be seen in as little as eight weeks of daily meditation.

With all of these benefits, it only makes sense to take up a daily practice of meditation/mindfulness. So how do you get started?

After thirty years of daily meditation practice, we have come to know that all the different techniques will eventually get you to the same place. The techniques are not the meditation; the silenced mind is the meditation. The techniques are just a means by which to achieve the silence.

Let's look at the different methods and techniques of meditation. There are meditations that are done while moving and others that are done just sitting in one place. As we go through these, remember that all the different types of meditation are really about silencing the chatter of the mind, so you might want to try different methods and pick the method that works best for you.

- *Tai Chi* is a moving meditation, one of the oldest forms of Chinese martial arts. It is a set of prearranged movements that are performed in slow motion. Once the movements have been memorized, it allows you to relax and focus on the feeling of the movement. Eventually, with practice, all other thoughts will cease.

- *Yoga* is another form of more active meditation with its origins in India. It combines movement and static poses, depending on what type of yoga is being practiced. In this way, it is similar to Tai Chi. As you hold and focus on the poses, all other thoughts will drop away.

- *Qi gong* (pronounced "chee gong") is a form of Chinese meditation that holds and focuses on static postures—similar to yoga.

- *Mantra meditation* is a common type of meditation, in which you focus and repeat a word, preferably a nonsensical word, over and over either out loud or silently. After some time, the word will drop away, leaving your mind in silence. This was one of the first meditations to become popular in the West. It was made famous by way of Transcendental Meditation (TM). Maharishi Mahesh Yogi brought it to the West, and it became popular because the band the Beatles was practicing it. The Maharishi thought this was a great type of meditation for Westerners because it was easier than some other types of meditation.

- *Breathing meditation* is the meditation most practiced world-wide. This is exactly what the name implies. You focus on your breath until even the breath is unnoticeable and you have the silenced mind. We will go more into the actual technique in just a moment.
- *Awareness/mindfulness* meditation is a type of meditation based on being in the present moment and being aware of the chatter that goes on in our minds. You become the observer of your thoughts. More on this, also, in a few moments.

One of the biggest misconceptions about meditation is that you need to attend some type of class or retreat, or that you need a teacher in order to do these meditations. However, after having taken many classes and courses over the past thirty years, we can honestly say that a course is not needed; you just need to sit and do the technique, and the results will come. We want to focus on a few of these techniques and save you the trouble by making them easy to understand and apply with minimal effort, so you can put them into practice. Someone can tell you how to meditate, but, until you experience it for yourself, you will never understand, and it will be just words and theory. It is like trying to tell a blind person what the sun is like or describing what chocolate is like to a person who has never tasted it. In other words, meditation goes beyond description; it is experiential.

## Breathing Meditation

The first of the meditations we want to start with is the breathing meditation. This is the most common meditation worldwide. As with any meditation, you can do this at any time—whether you are walk-ing, doing housework, or any other activity, but it is always easier to start in a quiet spot sitting still. So, find a nice quiet place to sit where you won't be interrupted. (Unless you are unable to sit, it is better not to try lying down. If you try to meditate lying down, you will more than likely fall asleep, and sleep is not meditating.) Assume a comfortable position; you do not need to sit in a "lotus position" unless that is how you are comfortable. Sitting in a nice comfortable chair, preferably with a straight back, is best. Sit with your feet on the floor and your hands on your thighs.

Next, close your eyes and become aware of your breath; just be aware of your breath going in and out. You can place your attention on your nostrils and focus on the breath flowing in and out of your nose. Or you can just be aware and follow the breath down to the bottom of your lungs and then back up and out of your nose. You may find it easier to focus on your nostrils and the feeling of the air going in and out. One point to remember is to allow the breath to be natural without changing the length or rate of your breathing—you want it to happen without effort. Many people will think this is too easy, that there must be more to it than this. Though this sounds simple, that doesn't make it easy. Most of us are so used to having this constant chatter of the mind that, at first, you may think you can't do it, or you may become frustrated while trying to do it.

As you become aware of the breath, your mind will likely wander to one thought, then to another, and maybe even another. First, you may think what you want to eat, then that may lead you to think about your favorite restaurant, then you may think of a birthday that you spent at that restaurant. All of these thoughts may come before you even realize that you have stopped being aware of your breathing. This is okay and natural, so do not let it upset you; just go back to being aware of the breath. When you notice the thoughts that arise, do not judge the thoughts; just let them go. Many people in meditation classes will become afraid in the middle of meditating because they have never experienced a silencing of the mind. So, it shocks them when the chatter disappears, and it causes them to open their eyes and stop the meditation. This is something to be aware of and to not let scare you.

Eventually, you will welcome the total silence. In this silence, there is a nothingness, which is actually a great peacefulness. You may not reach this state at the beginning, or every time you meditate, but the more you practice, the better you become. It is like learning any type of new skill—the more you practice, the better you get and the more natural it becomes. Over time and with practice, it will happen more naturally during all times and aspects of your life, and you will be able to do it even in the noisiest and busiest of times and places.

One note is that, when you start meditating, you are using your attention and focus, which is actually a form of tension. Concentration and focus are not meditation, but they are the tools to get there. This is only when you are beginning to practice; eventually, the attention changes to an awareness. This is why it is best to start in a quiet spot—when you have your attention on one thing, you exclude everything else. As your attention turns to awareness, you can do this at just about any time of the day, while you are going about your daily life.

## Awareness/Mindfulness Meditation

The second meditation we want to focus on is awareness/mindfulness meditation. Like the breathing meditation, it is easiest to begin in a quiet spot where you're not likely to be disturbed. Assume the same position as the breathing meditation: sitting in a straight-backed chair, feet on the floor, hands on your thighs. Quiet your mind and see if you can notice each individual thought. Once you become aware of the thoughts that come into your mind, observe them as if you are someone else watching, an outsider observing your thoughts. Once you become aware of the thought, let it go without any judgment, then become aware of the next thought, and then again, knowing that it is there and letting it go, like identifying it and putting each one into a river and watching it flow downstream. It's important with mindfulness meditation to keep your awareness open to any thought that may pop into your mind. You may have thoughts of past events, fears, or thoughts about the future, but no matter what it is, once you are aware of the thought, just let it go. As you continue with the practice, you will notice that you are not having these thoughts as much, and that being aware of the thought releases it, and that you are now simply in the moment without thoughts (as with the breathing meditation practice).

## How Long Should I Meditate?

How much time should you meditate? There is not a perfect amount of time of meditating. Some people will feel great at twenty minutes, and other people may choose to meditate for an hour. If you are just starting, five minutes may seem like a long time, so you may want to start with two minutes at a time and try this once or twice during the day. This may be all you can start with, and that's okay—you can work your way up to five minutes, then to ten minutes, to fifteen minutes, and then to twenty minutes. Once you reach the silenced mind, time seems to change: forty minutes will feel like just a few minutes.

## What Time of Day Is Best?

What time of the day should you meditate? The time of day does not matter. Any time you can make time is great, but many people find it easier to meditate first thing in the morning before the challenges of the day happen.

## Box Breathing

Box breathing is not a meditation in a traditional sense, but it is a great technique to use for calming the mind and the nervous system. It is used by US Navy Seals, athletes, and police officers in times of stress.

The method is simple. Just think of the four sides of a box:
- Side 1: Slowly inhale for 4–6 seconds
- Side 2: Hold the inhale for 4–6 seconds
- Side 3: Slowly exhale for 4–6 seconds
- Side 4: Hold the exhale for 4–6 seconds
- Repeat for as many cycles as desired.

You can increase the cycle as it becomes less challenging. Typically, after some practice, six seconds per side is a better length of time.

Breathing slowly this way allows for a build-up of $CO_2$ in the blood. Increased $CO_2$ allows for more oxygen to be released from the red blood cells, improving oxygenation throughout the body.

This breathing technique is great for improving and reducing stress. You can also use this technique at the beginning of a meditation session to help calm and clear your mind. A good way to begin is to perform ten cycles of box breathing before you start your meditation.

## Takeaways from Meditation

1. Meditation reduces stress and lowers cortisol levels.

2. Meditation increases the areas of the brain involved in learning, cognition, and emotional control. Changes can be seen in as few as eight weeks of daily meditation.

3. Start with sitting in a quiet place for five minutes, working up to twenty minutes, and just notice the thoughts that come into your mind. Keep it simple!

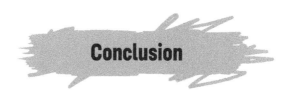

# Conclusion

The COVID-19 pandemic has opened our eyes to the endemic risks of an unhealthy lifestyle, obesity, and underlying health conditions. It's more important now than ever for us to understand some of the most important factors behind the silent epidemic of inflammation and inflammatory disease—stress, anti-aging hormones, our microbiome, and toxic dietary and environmental influences.

We hope that you find the information we provided here to be a jump start to eliminate these risks in your life. We've outlined a relatively comprehensive plan of integrating wellness into your everyday routine. In this program, all of us can find things that we need to implement or change.

However, we want to encourage you that small changes can and will make a big difference, so don't get overwhelmed. Even small changes and day-to-day consistency can allow us to experience much more energy and overall life satisfaction.

Best of luck to you in obtaining your optimal health and wellness!

# Appendix A

## Food and Fitness Journal

Studies show that keeping track of what you eat and your activity level is one of the most powerful tools to help you shed unwanted pounds and keep them off.

Use this food and fitness journal to help keep you working toward your goals.

| Breakfast | Serving | Calories |
|---|---|---|
| | | |
| | | |
| | | |

Total

| Mid-Morning Snack | Serving | Calories |
|---|---|---|
| | | |
| | | |
| | | |

Total

| Lunch | Serving | Calories |
|---|---|---|
| | | |
| | | |
| | | |

Total

Mid-Afternoon Snack

| | Serving | Calories |
|---|---|---|
| | | |
| | | |
| | | |

_____
Total

Dinner

| | Serving | Calories |
|---|---|---|
| | | |
| | | |
| | | |

_____
Total

Evening Snack

| | Serving | Calories |
|---|---|---|
| | | |
| | | |
| | | |

_____
Total

_____
Total Calories

Activity

| | Serving | Calories |
|---|---|---|
| | | |
| | | |
| | | |

_____
Total

_____
Total Calories Burned

# Appendix B

# Eating Plan "Laws"/Major Rules to Follow

**Rule #1:** Stay away from PUFA—eliminate PUFA from your diet!

**Rule #2:** There is not ONE diet that is perfect for everyone!

**Rule #3:** Create a "Do NOT Eat" list—read labels.

**Rule #4:** Eat ENOUGH calories—take in a healthy amount of proteins/fats/carbs for your situation.

**Rule #5:** Create a "What I CAN Eat" list—incorporate all three macronutrients (proteins/fats/carbs) into your daily meal plans.

**Rule #6:** Target for protein to be 10–35% of your daily caloric intake with at least 4 oz of protein with each meal.

**Rule #7:** Incorporate SFAs/MUFAs as your primary fat source.

**Rule #8:** A good goal for more sustainable weight loss over time is a target of one-half to one pound of weight loss per week.

**Rule #9:** It only takes twenty-one days to see noticeable improvements from dietary changes.

**Rule #10:** A healthy diet MUST be sustainable—think "paleo with a twist."

# Appendix C

## Dietary Options Chart

**Calories:** Men should aim for 2,600 calories/day. Women—2,000 calories/day.

| Total Intake | Men: 2,600 calories/day | Percentage | Men: 2,600 calories/day | Percentage |
|---|---|---|---|---|
| **Carbs** (4 cal/g) | 214.5 gms/day | 33% | 325 gms/day | 50% |
| **Fat** (9 cal/g) | 95 gms/day | 33% | 72 gms/day | 25% |
| **Protein** (4 cal/g) | 221 gms/day | 34% | 162.5 gms/day | 25% |

**Note:** 100 gms of protein is essentially equivalent two 6.0 oz servings of meat/day

| Total Intake | Women: 2,000 calories/day | Percentage | Women: 2,000 calories/day | Percentage |
|---|---|---|---|---|
| **Carbs** (4 cal/g) | 165 gms/day | 33% | 250 gms/day | 50% |
| **Fat** (9 cal/g) | 73 gms/day | 33% | 56 gms/day | 25% |
| **Protein** (4 cal/g) | 170 gms/day | 34% | 125 gms/day | 25% |

**Note:** Percentages may vary depending on person's preference. Low or no carb diets not recommended.
- 1 gm carbohydrate = 4 calories
- 1 gm fat = 9 calories
- 1 gm protein = 4 calories

## Beneficial Foods for a Pro-metabolic Diet

- Grass-fed meat
- Liver
- Wild-caught fish
- Oysters and other shellfish (high in zinc/selenium)
- Dairy products—including milk, cheese, yogurt, and cottage cheese
- Fruits/fruit juices
- Root vegetables—beets, carrots, potatoes (white/sweet)
- Green vegetables—preferably cooked
- Healthy fats—including animal fats (tallow), butter, coconut oil, olive oil, avocado oil
- Limit grain products that are not organic

## Phase 1: Eating Plan

- **Eat enough calories** to heal and increase your metabolism.
- A good description on how to eat would be **"paleo with a twist,"** meaning a diet based on:
    - Eating primarily unprocessed, unpackaged (ideally, organic) foods, consisting of dairy, meats, and vegetables.
    - Including starchy root vegetables and plenty of fruit. Don't be afraid of carbs—they are not the problem.
    - The number one rule is to **avoid PUFA (vegetable and seed/nut oils)**
    - Including saturated fats such as animal fat, butter, and/or coconut oil, or the monounsaturated fats such as olive and avocado oil.
- If, after twenty-one days, you are not feeling great or continue to have symptoms such as hormonal symptoms, GI/digestion problems, joint/muscle pain, or autoimmune conditions, then move to Phase 2.

## Phase 2: GI Healing Plan

The goal is limit the amount of undigested food that reaches the large intestine, which will limit the amount of endotoxin produced by the "bad" bacteria.

## Days 1–3

- Eat carbs, protein, and fat, but we are going to focus on the carbs in the easy-to-digest forms that will not reach the large intestine
- This will mainly be ripe fruit and fruit juices without the pulp.
- Easy-to-digest carbs will be foods such as mashed potatoes, rice, and processed flour products (do not eat cooled and reheated starches—cooling and reheating causes these to become resistant starches).

## After Day 3

- Start adding in other easily digestible carbs, preferably one at a time, to see if each particular food gives a reaction.
- Add a carrot salad once per day to help eliminate the endotoxin.

# Appendix D

## Supplement Chart

| Supplement | Benefits | Dosage | Timing | With or Without Food |
|---|---|---|---|---|
| **Vitamin B1** | Co-factor and increases cellular energy | 50–100 mg/day | AM | With |
| **Vitamin B2** | Co-factor and increases cellular energy | 2–5 mg/day | AM | With |
| **Vitamin B3** (as niacinamide) | Co-factor and increases cellular energy | 100 mg/day | AM | With |
| **Vitamin B5** | Co-factor and increases cellular energy | 50 mg/day | AM | With |
| **Vitamin B6** | Co-factor and increases cellular energy | 10 mg/day | AM | With |
| **Biotin** | Strong nails, hair growth, co-factor and increase in cellular energy | 1-3 mg/day | AM | With |
| **Folate** | Increase in cellular energy, healthy RBC production, prevention of birth defects | 500-1,000 mcg/day | AM | With |

| Vitamin A | Strengthens immune system, improves vision and reproductive function | 3,000-10,000 IU/day | AM | With |
|---|---|---|---|---|
| Vitamin D | Necessary for strong immune function, strong bones, calcium absorption and heart health | 5,000 IU/day | AM | With |
| Vitamin E | Necessary for strong immune function, reproductive function and hormone production and heart health | 50-100 IU/day | AM | With |
| Vitamin K (mk-4) | Important for clotting function, building strong bones and healthy hormone production | 1 mg/day | PM | With |
| Calcium | Key nutrient for overall health/ wellness | 800-1,400 mg/day | PM | Without |
| Magnesium | Key nutrient for overall health/ wellness, important for muscle relaxation, adequate thyroid function, for normal blood pressure, converting food into energy | 400–600 mg/day | PM | Without |

| | | | | |
|---|---|---|---|---|
| **Selenium** | Anti-cancer, anti-viral functions and important for strong immune system | 200-400 mcg/day | PM | Without |
| **Zinc** | Important for strong immune system | 10-20 mg/day | PM | Without |
| **Copper** | Important for nerve cell function, collagen formation and depleted by zinc | 1-2 mg/day | PM | Without |

# Appendix E

## Sleep Log

Use this sleep diary to record the quality and quantity of your sleep; your use of medicines, alcohol, and caffeinated drinks; and how you feel during the day.

**Fill out before going to bed**

| | | | | | | | |
|---|---|---|---|---|---|---|---|
| Today's date | | | | | | | |
| Number of caffeinated drinks and time I had them | | | | | | | |
| Number of alcoholic drinks and time I had them | | | | | | | |
| Naptimes and lengths | | | | | | | |
| Exercise times and lengths | | | | | | | |
| On a scale of 1–4, how sleepy did I feel today?<br>1—So sleepy I struggled to stay awake<br>2—Somewhat tired<br>3—Fairly alert<br>4—Awake and alert | | | | | | | |

## Fill out in the morning

| Today's date | | | | | | | |
|---|---|---|---|---|---|---|---|
| • Time I went to bed<br>• Time I got out of bed this morning<br>• Hours spent in bed | | | | | | | |
| Number of awakenings and total time awake | | | | | | | |
| How long it took to fall asleep | | | | | | | |
| Medicines taken before bed | | | | | | | |
| On a scale of 1–3, how alert did I feel when I woke up?<br>1—Alert<br>2—Alert but still tired<br>3—Sleepy | | | | | | | |

# Appendix F

# Resources for Excercise

*Sweat: Fitness App for Women*, app, v. 6.24.1 (December 2021), The Bikini Body Training Company Pty Ltd., iPhone iOs 13.0 or later. https://apps.apple.com/us/app/sweat-fitness-app-for-women/id1049234587#?platform=iphone

*V Shred: Nutrition and Fitness*, app, v. 2.3.6 (January 2022), V Shred LLC, iPhone iOs 12.1 or later. https://apps.apple.com/us/app/v-shred-diet-fitness/id1442111093

*One and Done Workout* by Meredith Shirk, fitness program, Meredith Shirk, Svelte Media, Inc. (2022). https://go.riseworkouts.com/7-minutes-a-day/?source=GOOGLEREMARKETING&offer_id=52&ep=322&tid=join1&ADID=431270358362&gclid=CjwKCAiA0KmPBhBqEiwAJqKK4_k2Oxl5GWrKhVO5ZsJnsFt-9NmjwNIXe_P7aQ4QYGptpM79txJu1kRoCqi4QAvD_BwE

*Beachbody Yoga Studio*, fitness program, Beachbody, LLC. (2022).https://www.beachbodyondemand.com/programs/beachbody-yoga-studio/start-here?referralprogramid

*Classes/Video on Demand*, yoga videos, Sunstone Yoga, LLC. (2021). https://www.sunstonefit.com/classes/video-on-demand

*ATHLEAN-X*, YouTube channel, Jeff Cavaliere, joined 2006 (latest: 2022). https://www.youtube.com/c/athleanx/featured

# Notes

## Introduction

1. University of Missouri-Columbia, "Intelligence can Link to Health and Aging," *ScienceDaily* (May 2019). https://www.sciencedaily.com/releases/2019/05/190508134509.htm

2. Liu, Chen, Gasparrini, & Kan, "Ambient Particulate Air Pollution and Daily Mortality in 652 Cities," *The New England Journal of Medicine*, vol. 381 no. 8 (August 2019): 705-715. https://www.nejm.org/doi/pdf/10.1056/NEJMoa1817364

## Part I: The Basics

### Chapter 1: Stress

1. James Brumley, "The 15 All-Time Best-Selling Prescription Drugs," *Kiplinger* (December 2017). https://www.kiplinger.com/slideshow/investing/t027-s001-the-15-all-time-best-selling-prescription-drugs/index.html

2. Centers for Disease Control and Prevention, "What is Prediabetes?" last reviewed December 21, 2021. https://www.cdc.gov/diabetes/basics/prediabetes.html#:~:text=Approximately%2096%20million%20American%20adults,%2C%20heart%20disease%2C%20and%20stroke

3. University of Missouri-Columbia, "Intelligence can Link to Health and Aging."

4. University of Missouri-Columbia, "Intelligence can Link to Health and Aging."; Brumley, "The 15 All-Time Best-Selling Prescription Drugs.";; Sarah Graham, "High Stress Levels Linked to Cellular Aging," *Scientific American*, (November 2004). https://www.scientificamerican.com/article/high -stress-levels-linked/

5. Roundtable on Environmental Health Sciences, Research, and Medicine; Board on Population Health and Public Health Practice; Institute of Medicine, "The Challenge: Chemicals in Today's Society," in Identifying and Reducing Environmental Health Risks of Chemicals in Our Society (Washington, DC: National Academies Press, 2014); and Business Wire, "The $72 Billion Weight Loss & Diet Control Market in the US, 2019-2023. Why Meal Replacements are Still Booming, but Not OTC Diet Pills," AP News (February 2019). https://apnews.com/press-release/business-wire/business-lifestyle-health-united-states-ec35f-3315f9a4816985615391f41815a

6. Ibid.

7. Oliver Milman, "US Cosmetics are Full of Chemicals Banned by Europe — Why?" The Guardian (May 2019). https://www.theguardian.com/us-news/2019/may/22/chemicals -in-cosmetics -us-restricted-eu

8. American Sleep Apnea Association, "Sleep Health," sleephealth.org (2017). https://www.sleephealth.org/sleep-health/the -state-of -sleephealth-in-america/

9. Aaron Kandola and Alina Sharon, "What is Chronic Stress and What are its Common Health Impacts?" Medical News Today (January 2022). https://www.medicalnewstoday.com/articles/323324

## Chapter 2: Hormones Overview

1. Oxford Dictionary, "hormone," Lexico Online Resource (2020).

2. "The Lower Your Cortisol Levels, the Younger You Look," April 24, 2017, Scientific Studies forum; R. Noordam, D.A. Gunn, C.C. Tomlin, M.P. Rozing, et al., "Cortisol Serum Levels in Familial Longevity and Perceived Age: The Leiden Longevity Study," Psychoneuroendocrinology, vol. 37, issue 10 (October 2012).

## Chapter 3: Cortisol and Adrenaline

1. Donald Young, "Glucocorticoid Action on Rat Thymus Cells," The Journal of Biological Chemistry, vol. 244, no. 8 (April 1968). https://www.jbc.org/article/S0021-9258(18)94385-1/pdf

## Chapter 4: Estrogen, Progesterone, and Testosterone

1.  James P. Grantham and Maciej Henneberg, "The Estrogen Hypothesis of Obesity," *PLoS One* (June 2014). https://pubmed. ncbi.nlm.nih.gov/24915457/

2.  N.C. Lee, et al., *Estrogen Therapy and the Risk of Breast, Ovary and Endometrial Cancer, in Aging, Reproduction, and the Climacteric* (NY & London: Plenum Press, 1986).

3.  T. L. Bush, et al., "Estrogen Use and All-Cause Mortality: Preliminary Results from the Lipid Research Clinics Program Follow-Up Study," *JAMA* (February 1983). https://pubmed.ncbi. nlm.nih.gov/6823043/

4.  N.C. Lee, et al., *Estrogen Therapy and the Risk of Breast, Ovary and Endometrial Cancer, in Aging, Reproduction, and the Climacteric.*

5.  Wikipedia, "Women's Health Initiative," last modified September 24, 2021. https://en.wikipedia.org/wiki/Women%27s_Health_Ini tiative

6.  Ray Peat Forum, "Birth Control Pills Increase Suicide Risk by More Than 300%." (December 2017). https://raypeatforum.com/ community/threads/birth-control-bc-pills-increase-suicide-risk-by-more-than-300.21340/; Morch, Skovlund, Hannaford, Iversen, Fielding, & Lidegaard, "Contemporary Hormonal Contraception and the Risk of Breast Cancer," *The New England Journal of Medicine* (December 2017). https://www.nejm.org/ doi/full/10.1056/nejmoa1700732; Kate Sheridan, "Breast Cancer: Birth Control May Increase Risk by Up to 38%," *Newsweek* (December 2017). https://www.newsweek.com/breast-cancer-birth-control-may-increase-risk-38-percent-736039; and Surabhi Dangi-Garimella, "The Final Word is Out: Menopausal HRT Triples the Risk of Breast Cancer," *AJMC* (July 2016). https://www. ajmc.com/view/molecular-profiling-identifies-potential-prog-nostic-biomarker-for-treatment-response-in-hnscc

7.  M. Akerlund, S. Batra, G. Helm, "Comparison of Plasma and Myometrial Tissue Concentrations of Estradiol-17 Beta and Progesterone in Nonpregnant Women," *Contraception* (April 1981). https://pubmed.ncbi.nlm.nih.gov/7273763/

8. Ibid.

9. C. Vermeulen-Meiners, L.J.Benedek Jaszmann, A.A. Haspels, J. Poortman, et al., "The Endogenous Concentration of Estradiol and Estrone in Normal Human Postmenopausal Endometrium," *Journal of Steroid Biochemistry*, vol. 21, issue 5 (1984). https://www.sciencedirect.com/science/article/abs/pii/0022473184903388

10. Akerlund, et al., "Comparison of Plasma and Myometrial Tissue Concentrations of Estradiol-17 Beta and Progesterone in Nonpreg- nant Women."

11. H. Kaunitz and C. A. Slanetz, and W. B. Atkinson, "Estrogen Response and Pigmentation of the Uterus in Vitamin E-Deficient Rat," *Proc. Soc. Exp. Biol. Med.* (1948). https://pubmed.ncbi.nlm.nih.gov/18112792/

12. M.J. Toth, A. Tchernof, C.K. Sites, E.T. Poehlman, "Effects of Menopuasal Status on Body Composition and Abdominal Fat Distribution," *Int. J. Obes. Relat. Metab. Disord.* (February 2000). https://pubmed.ncbi.nlm.nih.gov/10702775/

13. B.D. Greenstein, E.F. de Bridges, F.T. Fitzpatrick, "Aromatase Inhibitors Regenerate the Thymus in Aging Male Rats," *International Journal of Immunopharmacology*, vol. 14, issue 4 (May 1992): 541-553. https://pubmed.ncbi.nlm.nih.gov/1521922/

14. Ibid.

15. Tristan M. Nicholson and William A. Ricke, "Androgens and Estrogens in Benign Prostatic Hyperplasia: Past, Present, and Future," *Differentiation* (November 2011). https://pubmed.ncbi.nlm.nih.gov/21620560/

16. Grantham and Henneberg, "The Estrogen Hypothesis of Obesity."

17. N.C. Lee, et al., *Estrogen Therapy and the Risk of Breast, Ovary and Endometrial Cancer, in Aging, Reproduction, and the Climacteric.*

18. Ray Peat, "Aging, Estrogen, and Progesterone," accessed January 6, 2022, http://raypeat.com/articles/aging/aging-estrogen-pro-gester one.shtml

19. Anne Harding, "Men's Testosterone Levels Declined in Last 20 Years," *Reuter's Health* (January 2007). https://www.reute rs.com/article/health-testosterone-levels-dc-idUKKIM1697632 0061101?edtion -redirect=uk

20. Spencer Michels, "What is Biohacking and Why Should We Care?" *PBS News Hour* (September 2014). https://www.pbs.org/ newshour/science/biohacking-care

## Chapter 5: Insulin

1. Molecular Diversity Preservation International, *Nutrients*, (Basel, Switzerland: MDPI Publishing, 2009).

2. Haidut, "Baking Soda May Treat Cancer, Metformin May Cause It," *To Extract Knowledge from Matter* (May 2019). http://haidut.me/?p=171

3. G. Boden, "Free Fatty Acids, Insulin Resistance, and Type 2 Diabetes Mellitus," *Proc. Assoc. Am. Physicians* (May-June 1999). https://pubmed.ncbi.nlm.nih.gov/10354364/; and G. Boden, "Effects of Free Fatty Acids (FFA) on Glucose Metabolism: Significance for Insulin Resistance and Type 2 Diabetes," *Exp. Clin. Endocrinol Diabetes* (May 2003). https://pubmed.ncbi.nlm. nih.gov/12784183/

4. A.F. Whereat, F.E. Hull, M.W. Orishimo, "The Role of Succinate in the Regulation of Fatty Acid Synthesis by Heart Mitochondria," *J. Biol. Chem.* (September 1967). https://pubmed.ncbi.nlm.nih. gov/ 4383531/; P.J. Randle, P.B. Garland, C.N. Hales, & E.A. Newsholme, "The Glucose Fatty-Acid Cycle. Its Role in Insulin Sensitivity and the Metabolic Disturbances of Diabetes Mellitus," *Lancet* (April 1963). doi: 10.1016/s0140-6736(63)91500-9; Wikipedia, "Randle Cycle," last modified November 9, 2021. https://en.wikipedia.org/wiki/Randle_cycle; Antonio Blanco and Gustavo Blanco, "Integration and Regulation of Metabolism," in *Medical Biochemistry* (Academic Press, 2017); and Tara Dall, Dawn Thiselton, & Stephen Varvel, "Targeting Insulin Resistance: The Ongoing Paradigm Shift in Diabetes Prevention," *Evidence-Based Diabetes Management*, vol. 19, issue SP2 (March/April 2013). https://www.ajmc.com/view/targeting-insulin-resistance-the-on-going-paradigm-shift-in-diabetes-prevention

5. K.L. Hoen, N. Turner, et al., "Acute or Chronic Upregulation of Mitochondrial Fatty Acid Oxidation has No Net Effect on Whole Body Energy Expenditure or Adiposity," *Cell Metab.* (January 2010). doi: 10.1016/j.cmet.2009.11.008

6. Boden, "Effects of Free Fatty Acids (FFA) on Glucose Metabolism: Significance for Insulin Resistance and Type 2 Diabetes."

7. G. Boden, "Free Fatty Acids, Insulin Resistance, and Type 2 Diabetes Mellitus," *Proc. Assoc. Am. Physicians* (May–June 1999). https://pubmed.ncbi.nlm.nih.gov/10354364/

8. Heather Zeiger, "Mitochondria Function Changes as We Age," *Medical Xpress* (September 2015). https://medicalxpress.com/news/2015-09-mitochondrial-function-age.html

## Chapter 6: Thyroid Hormones

1. Xuefeng Ma, Shousheng Lie, Jie Zeng, Mengzhen Dong, Yifen Wang, Mengke Wang, & Yongning Xin, "Proportion of NAFLD Patients with Normal ALT Value in Overall NAFLD Patients: A Systematic Review and Meta-Analysis," *BMC Gastroenterol* (January 2020). doi: 10.1186/s12876-020-1165-z

2. J. Saxena, P.N. Singh, U. Srivastava, A.Q. Siddiqui, "A Study of Thyroid Hormones (t(3), t(4), & tsh) in Patients of Depression," *Indian Journal of Psychiatry* (July 2000). https://pubmed.ncbi.nlm.nih.gov/21407950/

3. Broda Barnes, *Hypothyroidism: The Unsuspected Illness* (Harper: 1976).

4. Saxena, et al., "A Study of Thyroid Hormones (t(3), t(4), & tsh) in Patients of Depression."

5. Barnes, Hypothyroidism: The Unsuspected Illness.

6. Ma, et al. , "Proportion of NAFLD Patients with Normal ALT Value in Overall NAFLD Patients: A Systematic Review and Meta-Analysis."

7. Healthline Editorial Team, "Forget 98.6 F. Humans are Cooling Off — Here's Why," *Healthline* (January 2020). https://www.healthline.com/health-news/forget-98-6-humans-now-have-lower-body-temperature-on-average-heres-why

8. Dennis Wilson, *Evidence-Based Approach to Restoring Thyroid Health* (Muskeegee Medical Publishing Company: 2014).

9. Lisa M. Coussens and Zena Werb, "Inflammation and Cancer," *Nature* (December 2002). doi:1038/nature01322

## Chapter 7: Inflammation

1. GBD 2017 Causes of Death Collaborators, "Global, Regional, and National Age-Sex-Specific Mortality for 282 Causes of Death in 195 Countries and Territories, 1980-2017: A Systematic Analysis for the Global Burden of Disease Study 2017," *The Lancet*, vol. 392, issue 10159 (November 2018). https://www.thelancet.com/journals/lancet/article/PIIS0140-6736(18)32203-7/fulltext

2. Ibid.

3. Mayo Clinic, "Metabolic Syndrome" (May 2021). https://www.mayoclinic.org/diseases-conditions/metabolic-syndrome/symptoms-causes/syc-20351916

4. Kimberly Amadeo, "Unemployment Rate by Year Since 1929 Compared to Inflation and GDP," *The Balance* (November 2021). https://www.thebalance.com/unemployment-rate-by-year-3305506; and Congressional Research Service, "Unemployment Rates During the COVID-19 Pandemic" (August 2021). https://sgp.fas.org/crs/misc/R46554.pdf

5. Michelle Crouch and Rachel Nania, "CDC Updates List of Underlying Conditions for Sever COVID-19," *AARP* (updated April 2021). https://www.aarp.org/health/conditions-treatments/info-2020/cdc-removes-covid-age-range-warning.html

6. Brent E. Wisse, "The Inflammatory Syndrome: The Role of Adipose Tissue Cytokines in Metabolic Disorders Linked to Obesity," *The Journal of the American Society of Nephrology* (November 2004). https://doi.org/10.1097/01.ASN.0000141966.69934.21

7. Crouch and Nania, "CDC Updates List of Underlying Conditions for Sever COVID-19."

8. Ibid.

9. Jessica Hamzelou, "Old Rt Brains Rejuvenated and New Neurons Grown by Asthma Drug," *New Scientist* (October 2015). https://

www.newscientist.com/article/dn28384-old-rat-brains-rejuve-nated-and-new-neurons-grown-by-asthma-drug/#; Mayo Clinic, "Metabolic Syndrome" (May 2021). https://www.mayoclinic.org/diseases-conditions/metabolic-syndrome/symptoms-causes/syc-20351916; and Lisa M. Coussens and Zena Werb, "Inflammation and Cancer," *Nature* (December 2002). doi: 10.1038/nature01322

10. A. Korniluk, O. Koper, H. Kemona, & V. Dymicka-Piekarska, "From Inflammation to Cancer," *Ir. J. Med. Sci.* (February 2017). doi: 10.1007/s11845-016-1464-0

11. Cancer Treatment Centers of America, "Inflammation Linked to Cancer, but Lifestyle Changes May Help" (August 2018). https://www.cancercenter.com/community/blog/2018/08/inflammation-linked-to-cancer-but-lifestyle-changes-may-help

12. Robert H. Shmerling, "Metabolic Syndrome is on the Rise: What It is and Why It Matters," *Health Harvard Publishing* (October 2020). https://www.health.harvard.edu/blog/metabolic-syndrome-is-on-the-rise-what-it-is-and-why-it-matters-2020071720621

13. Nathan S. Bryan, Dominik D. Alexander, James R. Coughlin, Andrew L. Milkwoski, Paolo Boffetta, "Ingested Nitrate and Nitrite and Stomach Cancer Risk: An Updated Review," *Food Chem Toxicol.* (October 2012). doi: 10.1016/j.fct.2012.07.062

## Chapter 8: Gastrointestinal Tract

1. Debora Mackenzie, "Bacteria Lurking in Blood Could Be Culprit in Countless Diseases," *NewScientist* (September 2016). https://www.newscientist.com/article/2104864-bacteria-lurking-in-blood-could-be-culprit-in-countless-diseases/

2. Maria Vazquez-Roque and Amy S. Oxentenko, "Nonceliac Gluten Sensitivity," *Mayo Clinic Proc.* (September 2015). https://pubmed.ncbi.nlm.nih.gov/26355401/

3. Centers for Disease Control and Prevention, "Who Gets Fungal Infections?" *CDC* (August 2021). https://www.cdc.gov/fungal/infections/index.html

4. C. Blanchaert, B. Strubbe, and H. Peeters, "Fecal Microbiota Transplantation in Ulcerative Colitis," *Acta Gastroenterol Belg.*

(October-December 2019). https://pubmed.ncbi.nlm.nih.gov/31 950808/

5. Benoit Chassaing, Omry Koren, Julia K. Goodrich, Angela C. Poole, et al., "Dietary Emulsifiers Impact the Mouse Gut Microbiota Promoting Colitis and Metabolic Syndrome," *Nature* (March 2015). https://pubmed.ncbi.nlm.nih.gov/25731162/

6. Ewen Callaway, "C-Section Babies are Missing Key Microbes," *Nature* (September 2019). https://www.nature.com/articles/ d41586-019-02807-x

7. Blanchaert, et al., "Fecal Microbiota Transplantation in Ulcerative Colitis."

8. (1d section 2, also in text). G.V. Mann, A. Spoerry, M. Gray, and D. Jarashow, "Atherosclerosis in the Masai," *Am. J. Epidemiol*, (January 1972). https://pubmed.ncbi.nlm.nih.gov/5007361/

9. Callaway, "C-Section Babies are Missing Key Microbes."

10. Ibid.

11. Warwick Selby, Paul Pavli, Brendan Crotty, Tim Florin, et al. "Two-Year Combination Antibiotic Therapy with Clarithromycin, Rifabutin, and Clofazimine for Crohn's Disease," *Gastroenterology* (June 2007). https://pubmed.ncbi.nlm.nih. gov/17570206/; and Niv Zmora, Gili Zilberman-Schapira, Jotham Suez, Zamir Halpern, et al., "Personalized Gut Mucosal Colonization Resistance to Empiric Probiotics is Associated with Unique Host and Microbiome Features," *Cell*, vol. 174, issue 6 (September 2018). https://www.cell.com/cell/fulltext/S0092-8674(18)311024?_returnURL=https%3A%2F%2Flinkinghub. elsevier.com%2Fretrieve%2Fpii%2FS0092867418311024%3F-showall%3Dtrue

12. Alan T. Tang, Katie R. Sullivan, Courtney C. Hong, Lauren M. Goddard, et al., "Distinct Cellular Roles for PDCD10 Define a Gut-Brain Axis in Cerebral Cavernous Malformation," *Sci. Transl. Med.* (November 2019). https://pubmed.ncbi.nlm.nih. gov/31776290/

13. Mackenzie, "Bacteria Lurking in Blood Could Be Culprit in Countless Diseases."

14. NYU School of Medicine, "Gut Bacteria Determine Speed of Tumor Growth in Pancreatic Cancer," *NYU* (March 2018). https://www.nyu.edu/about/news-publications/news/2018/march/gut-bacteria-determine-speed-of-tumor-growth-in-pancreatic-cance.html

15. Peter Christopher Konturek, Igor Alexander Harsch, Kathrin Konturek, Monic Schink, et al., "Gut-Liver Axis: How Do Gut Bacteria Influence the Liver?" *Medical Sciences* (September 2018). https://www.ncbi.nlm.nih.gov/pmc/articles/PMC6165386/

## Chapter 9: Endotoxin

1. Yoshinori Nagai and Kiyoshi Takatsu, "Role of the Immune System in Obesity-Associated Inflammation and Insulin Resistance," in *Nutrition in the Prevention and Treatment of Abdominal Obesity* (Academic Press, 2014); Richard L. Young, Amanda L. Lumsden, Alyce M. Martin, Gudrun Schober, et al., "Augmented Capacity for Peripheral Serotonin Release in Human Obesity," *International Journal of Obesity* (March 2018). https://pubmed.ncbi.nlm.nih.gov/29568107/; and Flinders University, "How Gut Bacteria Negatively Influences Blood Sugar Level," *Medical Press* (September 2019). https://medicalxpress.com/news/2019-09-gut-bacteria-negatively-blood-sugar.html

2. Chang Myung Oh, Sangkyu Park, & Hail Kim, "Serotonin as a New Therapeutic Target for Diabetes Mellitus and Obesity," *Diabetes Metab. Journal* (April 2016). https://pubmed.ncbi.nlm.nih.gov/27126880/

3. Mackenzie, "Bacteria Lurking in Blood Could Be Culprit in Countless Diseases."

4. Kelton Tremellen, Natalie McPhee, Karma Pearce, Sven Benson, et al., "Endotoxin-Initiated Inflammation Reduces Testosterone Production in Men of Reproductive Age," *American Journal of Physiology* (November 2017). https://pubmed.ncbi.nlm.nih.gov/29183872/

5. Kelton Tremellen, "Gut Endotoxin Leading to a Decline in Gonadal Function (GELDING): A Novel Theory for the Development of Late Onset Hypogonadism in Obese Men," *Basic*

*Clin. Androl.* (June 2016). https://www.ncbi.nlm.nih.gov/pmc/articles/PMC4918028/

6. Ziba Kashef, "The Enemy Within: Gut Bacteria Drive Autoimmune Disease," *YaleNews* (March 2018). https://news.yale.edu/2018/03/08/enemy-within-gut-bacteria-drive-autoimmune -disease

7. Tang, et al., "Distinct Cellular Roles for PDCD10 Define a Gut-Brain Axis in Cerebral Cavernous Malformation."

8. Chassaing, et al., "Dietary Emulsifiers Impact the Mouse Gut Microbiota Promoting Colitis and Metabolic Syndrome."

## Part II: Diets and Dieting

### Chapter 10: The Perfect Diet

1. Weston A. Price, "The Perfect Diet," in *Nutrition and Physical Degeneration* (Price-Potter Nutrition Foundation, 2009); and John Ikerd, "Americans: Overfed and Undernourished," *Small Farm Today* (March-April 2007). http://web.missouri.edu/~ikerdj/papers/SFT-Overfed%20-%20Undernourished.htm

### Chapter 11: It's All About Calories

1. Richard Conniff, "The Hunger Gains: Extreme Calorie-Restriction Diet Shows Anti-Aging Results," *Scientific American* (February 2017). https://www.scientificamerican.com/article/the-hunger-gains-extreme-calorie-restriction-diet-shows-anti-aging-results/

2. Stephan Guyenet, "The Body Fat Setpoint, Part IV: Changing the Setpoint," *Whole Health Source* (January 2010). http://wholehealthsource.blogspot.com/2010/01/body-fat-setpoint-part-iv-changing.html

3. Conniff, "The Hunger Gains: Extreme Calorie-Restriction Diet Shows Anti-Aging Results."

### Chapter 13: History of PUFA

1. Centers for Disease Control and Prevention, "Adult Obesity Facts," last reviewed September 30, 2021. https://www.cdc.gov/obesity/data/adult.html; and Wealth Daily, "Prevalence of Obesity

Among U.S. Adults Aged 20-74" [photo]. https://images.angel-pub.com/2015/19/30721/4.png

2. Chris A. Knobbe and Marija Stojanoska, "The 'Displacing Foods of Modern Commerce' are the Primary and Proximate Cause of Age-Related Macular Degeneration: A Unifying Singular Hypothesis," *Med Hyphotheses* (November 2017). https://pubmed.ncbi.nlm.nih.gov/29150284/

3. Ibid.

4. Ibid.

5. I.A. Prior, F. Davidson, C.E. Salmond, & Z. Czochanska, "Cholesterol, coconuts, and Diet on Polynesian Atolls: A Natural Experiment: The Pukapuka and Tokelau Island Studies," *Am. J. Clin. Nutr.* (August 1981). https://pubmed.ncbi.nlm.nih.gov/7270479/

## Chapter 14: Omega-6 ves. Omega-3—Which One is Worse?

1. B.S. Peskin, "Why Fish Oil Fails: A Comprehensive 21st Century Lipids-Based Physiologic Analysis," *J Lipids* (January 2014). https://pubmed.ncbi.nlm.nih.gov/24551453/

2. Reports and Data, "Fish Oil Market to Reach USD 5.42 Billion by 2026," *GlobeNewswire* (April 2019). https://www.globenewswire.com/news-release/2019/04/09/1799956/0/en/Fish-Oil-Market-To-Reach-USD-5-42-Billion-By-2026-Reports-And-Data.html

3. C.D. Malis, P.C. Weber, A. Leaf, & J.V. Bonventre, "Incorporation of Marine Lipids into Mitochondrial Membranes Increases Susceptibility to Damage by Calcium and Reactive Oxygen Species: Evidence for Enhanced Activation of Phospholipase A2 in Mitochondria Enriched with N-3 Fatty Acids," Proc. Natl. Acad. Sci. USA (November 1990). https://pubmed.ncbi.nlm.nih.gov/2123344/

4. Ibid.

5. Raquel Escrich, Irmgard Costa, Montserrat Moreno, Marta Cubedo, et al., "A high-corn-oil diet strongly stimulates mammary carcinogenesis, while a high-extra-virgin-olive-oil diet has a weak effect, through changes in metabolism, immune system function and proliferation/apoptosis pathways," in The Journal

of Nutritional Biochemistry, vol. 64 (Elsevier, 2019); James L. Miller, Magdalena Blaszkiewicz, Cordell Beaton, Cory P. Johnson, et al., "A Peroxidized Omega-3-Enriched Polyunsaturated Diet Leads to Adipose and Metabolic Dysfunction," in The Journal of Nutritional Biochemistry, vol. 64 (Elsevier, 2019); C.D. Malis, "Incorporation of Marine Lipids"; and R.K. Singh, R. W. Hardy, M. H. Wang, J. Williford, et al., "Stearate Inhibits Human Tumor Cell Invasion," Invasion Metastasis (1995). https://pubmed.ncbi.nlm.nih.gov/8621270/

6. Sanjeev Sethi, Ouliana Ziouzenkova, Heyu Ni, Denisa D. Wagner, et al., "Oxidized Omega-3 Fatty Acids in Fish Oil Inhibit Leukocyte-Endothelial Interactions Through Activation of PPAR Alpa," *Blood* (August 2002). https://pubmed.ncbi.nlm.nih.gov/12149216/

7. Saray Gutierrez, Sara L. Svahn, Maria E. Johansson, "Effects of Omega-3 Fatty Acids on Immune Cells," *Int. J. Mol. Sci.* (October 2019).

8. Raquel Escrich, Irmgard Costa, Montserrat Moreno, Marta Cubedo, et al., "A high-corn-oil diet strongly stimulates mammary carcinogenesis, while a high-extra-virgin-olive-oil diet has a weak effect, through changes in metabolism, immune system function and proliferation/apoptosis pathways," in *The Journal of Nutritional Biochemistry*, vol. 64 (Elsevier, 2019); Saray Gutierrez, Sara L. Svahn, Maria E. Johansson, "Effects of Omega-3 Fatty Acids on Immune Cells," *Int. J. Mol. Sci.* (October 2019); Antonella Mannini, Nadja Kerstin, Lido Calorini, Gabriele Mugnai, & Salvatore Ruggieri, "Dietary N-3 Polyunsaturated Fatty Acids Enhance Metastatic Dissemination of Murine T Lymphoma Cells," *Br. J. Nutr.* (October 2009). https://pubmed.ncbi.nlm.nih.gov/19785932/; Hillary L. Woodworth, Sarah J. McCaskey, David M. Duriancik, Jonathan F. Clinthorne, et al., "Dietary Fish Oil Alters T Lymphocyte Cell Populations and Exacerbates Disease in a Mouse Model of Inflammatory Colitis," *Cancer Res.* (October 2010). https://pubmed.ncbi.nlm.nih.gov/20798218/; Medical News Today, "Link between Fish Oil and Increased Risk of Colon Cancer in Mice" (October 2010). https://www.medicalnewstoday.com/mnt/releases/203683#1; M.B. Veierød, D.S. Thelle, & P. Laake,

"Diet and Risk of Cutaneous Malignant Melanoma: A Prospective Study of 50,575 Norwegian Men and Women," *Int. J. Cancer* (May 1997); Sanjeev Sethi, Ouliana Ziouzenkova, Heyu Ni, Denisa D. Wagner, et al., "Oxidized Omega-3 Fatty Acids in Fish Oil Inhibit Leukocyte-Endothelial Interactions Through Activation of PPAR Alpa," *Blood* (August 2002). https://pubmed.ncbi.nlm.nih.gov/12149216/; Francesca L. Crowen, Naomi E. Allen, Paul N. Appleby, Kim Overvad, et al., "Fatty Acid Composition of Plasma Phospholipids and Risk of Prostate Cancer in a Case-Control Analysis Nested Within the European Prospective Investigation into Cancer and Nutrition," *Am. J. Clin. Nutr.* (November 2008). https://pubmed.ncbi.nlm.nih.gov/18996872/; and Theodore M. Brasky, Amy K. Darke, Xiaoling Song, Catherine M. Tange, et al., "Plasma Phospholipid Fatty Acids and Prostate Cancer Risk in the SELECT Trial," *Journal of the National Cancer Institute*, vol. 105, issue 15 (August 2013). https://academic.oup.com/jnci/article/105/15/1132/926341

9.  S.G. Kaasgaard, G. Hølmer, C.E. Høy, W.A. Behrens, & J.L. Beare-Rogers, "Effects of Dietary Linseed Oil and Marine Oil on Lipid Peroxidation in Monkey Liver in Vivo and in Vitro," Lipids (October 1992). https://pubmed.ncbi.nlm.nih.gov/1435093/9. S.G. Kaasgaard, G. Hølmer, C.E. Høy, W.A. Behrens, & J.L. Beare-Rogers, "Effects of Dietary Linseed Oil and Marine Oil on Lipid Peroxidation in Monkey Liver in Vivo and in Vitro," Lipids (October 1992). https://pubmed.ncbi.nlm.nih.gov/1435093/

## Chapter 15: Stay away from PUFA

1.  M.R. L'Abbe, K.D. Trick, J.L. Beare-Rogers, "Dietary (N-3) Fatty Acids Affect Rat Heart, Liver and Aorta Protective Enzyme Activities and Lipid Peroxidation," J. Nutr. (September 1991). https://pubmed.ncbi.nlm.nih.gov/1880611/

2.  Sanjoy Ghosh, Girish Kewalramani, Gloria Yuen, Thomas Pulinilkunnil, et al., "Induction of Mitochondrial Nitrative Damage and Cardiac Dysfunction by Chronic Provision of Dietary Omega-6 Polyunsaturated Fatty Acids," Free Radic. Biol. Med. (November 2006). https://pubmed.ncbi.nlm.nih.gov/17023268/

3. Deccan Chronicle, "44% women are energy deficient" (September 2017) https://www.deccanchronicle.com/lifestyle/health-and-wellbeing/270917/44-per-cent-women-are-energy-deficient.html

4. T.L. Goodfried, D.L. Ball, H. Raff, E.D. Bruder, et al., "Oxidized Products of Linoleic Acid Stimulate Adrenal Steroidogenesis," Endocr. Res. (November 2002). https://pubmed.ncbi.nlm.nih.gov/12530633/; and Eric D. Bruder, Dennis L. Ball, Theodore L. Goodfried, & Hershel Raff, "An Oxidized Metabolite of Linoleic Acid Stimulated Corticosterone Production by Rat Adrenal Cells," Am. J. Physiol. Regul. Integr. Comp. Physiol. (June 2003). https://pubmed.ncbi.nlm.nih.gov/12689852/

5. J. Mertin and R. Hunt, "Influence of Polyunsaturated Fatty Acids on Survival of Skin Allografts and Tumor Incidence in Mice," Proceedings of the National Academy of Sciences, vol. 73 (March 1976). https://ur.booksc.eu/book/58494459/680934

6. H. Glauber, P. Wallace, K. Griver, & G. Brechtel, "Adverse Metabolic Effect of Omega-3 Fatty Acids in Non-Insulin-Dependent Diabetes Mellitus," Ann Intern Med. (May 1988). https://pubmed.ncbi.nlm.nih.gov/3282462/

7. Hillary L. Woodworth, Sarah J. McCaskey, David M. Duriancik, Jonathan F. Clinthorne, et al., "Dietary Fish Oil Alters T Lymphocyte Cell Populations and Exacerbates Disease in a Mouse Model of Inflammatory Colitis," Cancer Res. (October 2010). https://pubmed.ncbi.nlm.nih.gov/20798218/; and NHS Choices, "Diet 'causes bowel disease," NHS, and Nursing Times (July 2009). https://www.nursingtimes.net/news/behind-the-headlines-archive/diet-causes-bowel-disease-28-07-2009/

8. NHS Choices, "Diet 'causes bowel disease," NHS, and Nursing Times (July 2009). https://www.nursingtimes.net/news/behind-the-headlines-archive/diet -causes-bowel-disease-28-07-2009/

9. Hyung Wook Park, "Longevity, Aging, and Caloric Restriction: Clive Maine McCay and the Construction of a Multidisciplinary Research Program," Historical Studies in the Natural Sciences (Winter 2010). https://pubmed.ncbi.nlm.nih.gov/20514744/; and G. Durand and F. Desnoyers, "Polyunsaturated Fatty Acids and

Aging. Lipofuscins: Structure, Origin and Development," Ann. Nutr. Aliment (1980). https://pubmed.ncbi.nlm.nih.gov/7001991/

10. Yasushi Endo, Chieko Hayashi, Takashi Yamanaka, Koichi Takayose, et al., "Linolenic Acid as the Main Source of Acrolein Formed During Heating of Vegetable Oils," Journal of the American Oil Chemists' Society, vol. 90, issue 7 (September 2012). https://www.proquest.com/docview/1370420441; and K. Udeni Alwis, B. Rey deCastro, John C. Morrow, & Benjamin C. Blount, "Acrolein Exposure in US Tobacco Smokers and Non-Tobacco Users: NHANES 2005-2006," Environ. Health Perspect. (December 2015). https://www.ncbi.nlm.nih.gov/pmc/articles/PMC4671235/

11. Malis, et al., "Incorporation of Marine Lipids into Mitochondrial Membranes Increases Susceptibility to Damage by Calcium and Reactive Oxygen Species: Evidence for Enhanced Activation of Phospholipase A2 in Mitochondria Enriched with N-3 Fatty Acids."

12. Ibid.

13. E.V. McCollum, The Newer Knowledge of Nutrition (New York City: The MacMillan Company, 1918).

14. Ibid.

15. Poonamjot Deol, Jane R. Evans, Joseph Dhahbi, Karthikeyani Chellappa, et al., "Soybean Oil Is More Obesogenic and Diabetogenic than Coconut Oil and Fructose in Mouse: Potential Role for the Liver" (July 2015). https://journals.plos.org/plosone/article?id=10.1371/journal.pone.0132672#abstract0

16. C.D. Malis, et al., "Incorporation of Marine Lipids into Mitochondrial Membranes Increases Susceptibility to Damage by Calcium and Reactive Oxygen Species: Evidence for Enhanced Activation of Phospholipase A2 in Mitochondria Enriched with N-3 Fatty Acids."

17. Deol, et al., "Soybean Oil Is More Obesogenic and Diabetogenic than Coconut Oil and Fructose in Mouse: Potential Role for the Liver."

## Chapter 16: The Good Fat—Saturated Fat

1.  Arne Astrup, Faidon Magkos, Dennis M. Bier, J. Thomas Brenna, et al., "Saturated Fats and Health: A Reassessment and Proposal for Food-Based Recommendations," Journal of the American College of Cardiology, vol. 76, issue 7 (August 2020). https://www.science-direct.com/science/article/pii/S0735109720356874?via%3Dihub

2.  Zoë Harcombe, Julien S Baker, Stephen Mark Cooper, Bruce Davies, et al., "Evidence from Randomised Controlled Trials did not Support the Introduction of Dietary Fat Guidelines in 1977 and 1983: A Systematic Review and Meta-Analysis," Open Heart, vol. 2, issue 1 (February 2015). https://openheart.bmj.com/content/2/1/e000196

3.  Susan Scutti, "Does saturated Fat Clog Your Arteries? Controversial Paper Says 'No,'" CNN (April 2017). https://www.cnn.com/2017/04/25/health/saturated-fat-arteries-study/index.html

4.  E.R. Farnworth, J.K. Kramer, B.K. Thompson, & A.H. Corner, "Role of Dietary Saturated Fatty Acids on Lowering the Incidence of Heart Lesions in Male Rats," J. Nutr. (February 1982). https://pubmed.ncbi.nlm.nih.gov/7057261/

5.  Astrup, et al., "Saturated Fats and Health: A Reassessment and Proposal for Food-Based Recommendations."

6.  Ray Peat, "Fats, Functions, and Malfunctions," Ray Peat (2013). http://raypeat.com/articles/articles/fats-functions-malfunctions.shtml

7.  R.K. Singh, R. W. Hardy, M. H. Wang, J. Williford, et al., "Stearate Inhibits Human Tumor Cell Invasion," Invasion Metastasis (1995). https://pubmed.ncbi.nlm.nih.gov/8621270/

8.  A.A. Nanji, K. Jokelainen, G.L. Tipoe, A Rahemtulla, et al., "Dietary saturated fatty acids reverse inflammatory and fibrotic changes in rat liver despite continued ethanol administration," J. Pharmacol. Exp. Ther. (November 2001). https://pubmed.ncbi.nlm.nih.gov/11602676/

9.  Prior, et al., "Cholesterol, coconuts, and Diet on Polynesian Atolls: A Natural Experiment: The Pukapuka and Tokelau Island Studies."

10. Grigorov I.G., Kozlovskaia S.G., Semes'ko T.M., Asadov Sh.A., "Characteristics of Actual Nutrition of the Long-Lived Population of Azerbaijan," Vopr Pitan (1991).

## Part III: The Plan

### Diet Phase One: Eating Plan

1. Jules Bernstein, "America's Most Widely Consumed Oil Causes Genetic Changes in the Brain," UC Riverside News, (January 2020). https://news.ucr.edu/articles/2020/01/17/americas-most-wide-ly-consumed-oil-causes-genetic-changes-brain

2. Albert Tannenbaum and Herbert Silverstone, "Nutrition in Relation to Cancer," Advances in Cancer Research, vol. 1 (1953). https://www.sciencedirect.com/science/article/abs/pii/S0065230X08600093

3. Jack LaLanne, quote: "If man made it, don't eat it." https://www.chatelaine.com/health/fitness/10-things-we-learned-from-jack-lalanne/#:~:text=%E2%80%9CIf%20man%20made%20it%2C%20don,it%20in%20the%20first%20place.

4. (1d section 2, also in text); Mann, et al., "Atherosclerosis in the Masai."

5. Micah Dorfner, "Are You Getting Too Much Protein?" Mayo Clinic (February 2017). https://newsnetwork.mayoclinic.org/discussion/are-you-getting-too-much-protein/

6. (1d section 2, also in text). Mann, et al.,"Atherosclerosis in the Masai."

7. a. F. Lanfranco, L. Gianotti, A. Picu, R. Giordano, et al., "Effects of Free Fatty Acids on ACTH and Cortisol Secretion in Anorexia Nervosa," Eur. J. Endocrinol. (May 2006). https://pubmed.ncbi.nlm.nih.gov/16645021/; and Wikipedia, "Randle Cycle," last modified November 9, 2021. https://en.wikipedia.org/wiki/Randle_cycle

8. University of Aberdeen, "New Study Finds that Fat Consumption is the Only Cause of Weight Gain" (July 2018). https://www.abdn.ac.uk/news/12079/

9. Emily L. Goldberg, Irina Shchukina, Jennifer L. Asher, Sviatoslav Sidorov, et. al., "Ketogenesis Activates Metabolically Protective γδ T Cells in Visceral Adipose Tissue," Nat. Metab. (January 2020). https://pubmed.ncbi.nlm.nih.gov/32694683/

10. Ibid.

11. American Liver Foundation, "Nonalcoholic Fatty Liver Disease (NAFLD)," date accessed: January 11, 2022. https://liverfoundation.org/for-patients/about-the-liver/diseases-of-the-liver/non-alcoholic-fatty-liver-disease/#:~:text=About%20100%20million%20individuals%20in,over%20the%20past%2020%20years.

## Diet Phase Two: The GI Healing Plan

1. VIVO Pathophysiology, "Gastrointestinal Transit: How Long Does It Take?" *vivo.colostate.edu*, date accessed: January 11, 2022. http://www.vivo.colostate.edu/hbooks/pathphys/digestion/basics/transit.html

## Supplements

1. Institute of Medicine Committee, "Overview of Food Fortification in the United States and Canada," in *Dietary Reference Intakes: Guiding Principles for Nutrition Labeling and Fortification* (Washington: National Academies Press, 2003).

2. Sean Johnson and Shin-ichiro Imai, "NAD+ Biosynthesis, Aging, and Disease," published online (February 2018). doi: 10.12688/f1000research.12120.1; and Liana Roberts Stein and Shin-ichiro Imai, "The Dynamic Regulation of NAD Metabolism in Mitochondria," *Trends Endocrinol. Metab.* (July 2012). doi: 10.1016/j.tem.2012.06.005

3. Collin D. Heer, Daniel J. Sanderson, Yousef M.O. Alhammad, Mark S. Schmidt, et al., "Coronavirus Infection and PARP Expression Dysregulate the NAD Metabolome: A Potentially Actionable Component of Innate Immunity," *J. Biol. Chem.* (December 2020). https://pubmed.ncbi.nlm.nih.gov/33051211/

4. Michael B. Zimmermann, Rita Wegmuller Christophe Zeder, Nourredine Chaouki, et al., "The Effects of Vitamin A Deficiency

and Vitamin A Supplementation on Thryoid Function in Goitrous Children," *J. Clin. Endocrinol. Metab.* (November 2004). https://pubmed.ncbi.nlm.nih.gov/15531495/; and Michael B. Zimmermann, "Interactions of Vitamin A and Iodine Deficiencies: Effects on the Pituitary-Thyroid Axis," *Int. J. Vitam. Nutr. Res.* (May 2007). https://pubmed.ncbi.nlm.nih.gov/18214025/

5.  A.M. Kligman, O.H. Mills Jr., J.J. Leyden, P.R. Gross, et al., "Oral Vitamin A in Acne Vulgaris. Preliminary Report," *Int. J. Dermatol* (May 1981). https://pubmed.ncbi.nlm.nih.gov/6453848/

6.  M. Resasco, L. Canobbio, F. Trave, G. Valenti, et al., "Plasma Retinol Levels and Side Effects Following High-Dose Retinyl Acetate in Breast Cancer Patients," *Anticancer Res.* (November-December 1988). https://pubmed.ncbi.nlm.nih.gov/3218964/; A. Maiorana and P.M. Gullino, "Effect of Retinyl Acetate on the Incidence of Mammary Carcinomas and Hepatomas in Mice," *J. National Caner Inst.* (Mar 1980). https://pubmed.ncbi.nlm.nih.gov/6928249/; and David L. McCormick and Richard C. Moon, "Influence of Delayed Administration of Retinyl Acetate on Mammary Carcinogenesis," *Cancer Research* (July 1982). https://cancerres.aacrjournals.org/content/canres/42/7/2639.full.pdf

7.  McCormick and Moon, "Influence of Delayed Administration of Retinyl Acetate on Mammary Carcinogenesis" (1982). https://cancerres.aacrjournals.org/content/canres/42/7/2639.full.pdf; and S. Holtzman, "Retinyl Acetate Inhibits Estrogen-Induced Mammary Carcinogenesis in Female ACI Rats," *Carcinogenesis* (February 1988). https://pubmed.ncbi.nlm.nih.gov/3123084/

8.  F.P. Giraldi, A.G. Ambrogio, M. Andrioli, F. Sanguin, et al., "Potential Role for Retinoic Acid in Patients with Cushing's Disease," *J. Clin. Endocrinol Metab.* (October 2012). https://pubmed.ncbi.nlm.nih.gov/22851491/

9.  M.H. Iversen and R.G. Hahn, "Acute Effects of Vitamin A on the Kinetics of Endotoxin in Conscious Rabbits," *Intensive Care Med.* (October 1999). https://pubmed.ncbi.nlm.nih.gov/10551976/; and S.Y. Kim, J.E. Koo, M.R. Song, & J.Y. Lee, "Retinol Suppresses the Activation of Toll-Like Receptors in MyD88 and Stat1

Independent Manners," *Inflammation* (April 2013). https://pubmed.ncbi.nlm.nih.gov/23086657/

10. D. Bonhomme, V. Pallet, G. Dominguez, L. Servant, et al., "Retinoic Acid Modulates Intrahippocampal Levels of Corticosterone in Middle-Aged Mice: Consequences on Hippocampal Plasticity and Contextual Memory," *Frontiers in Aging Neuroscience*, vol. 6 (February 2014). https://www.ncbi.nlm.nih.gov/pmc/articles/PMC3917121/

11. Cynthia Aranow, "Vitamin D and the Immune System," *J. Investigative. Med.* (August 2011). https://pubmed.ncbi.nlm.nih.gov/21527855/

12. Jade Scipioni, "The Supplement Dr. Fauci Takes to Help Keep his Immune System Healthy," *CNBC* (September 2020). https://www.cnbc.com/2020/09/14/supplements-white-house-advisor-fauci-takes-every-day-to-help-keep-his-immune-system-healthy.html

13. "New Study: Vitamin D Reduces Risk of ICU Admission 97%," COVID.US.ORG (September 2020). https://covid.us.org/2020/09/03/new-study-vitamin-d-reduces-risk-of-icu-admission-97/

14. Sharon L. McDonnell, Carole A. Baggerly, Christine B.. French, Leo L. Baggerly, et al., "Breast cancer risk markedly lower with serum 25-hydroxyvitamin D concentrations ≥60 vs <20 ng/ml (150 vs 50 nmol/L): Pooled analysis of two randomized trials and a prospective cohort," *PLoS One* (June 2018). https://pubmed.ncbi.nlm.nih.gov/29906273/

15. Dimitrios T Papadimitriou, "The Big Vitamin D Mistake," *J. Prev. Med. Public Health* (July 2017). https://pubmed.ncbi.nlm.nih.gov/28768407/

16. R. Ricciarelli, P. Maroni, N. Ozer, J.M. Zingg, et al., "Age-Dependent Increase of Collagenase Expression Can Be Reduced by Alpha-Tocopherol Via Protein Kinase C Inhibition," *Free Radic. Biol. Med.* (October 1999). https://pubmed.ncbi.nlm.nih.gov/10515576/

17. G.C. Desjardins, A. Beaudet, H.M. Schipper, & J.R. Brawer, "Vitamin E Protects Hypothalamic Beta-Endorphin Neurons

from Estradiol Neurotoxicity," *Endocrinology* (November 1992). https://pubmed.ncbi.nlm.nih.gov/1425446/

18. M. Ciavatti and S. Renaud, "Oxidative Status and Oral Contraceptive. Its Relevance to Platelet Abnormalities and Cardiovascular Risk," *Free Radic. Biol. Med.* (1991). https://pubmed.ncbi.nlm.nih.gov/1855673/

19. F. Umeda, K. Kato, K. Muta, & H. Ibayashi, "Effect of Vitamin E on Function of Pituitary-Gonadal Axis in Male Rats and Human Subjects," *Endocrinol Jpn.* (1982). https://pubmed.ncbi.nlm.nih.gov/6816576/

20. Q. Jiang, I. Elson-Schwab, C. Courtemanche, & B.N. Ames, Gamma-Tocopherol and Its Major Metabolite, in Contrast to Alpha-Tocopherol, Inhibit Cyclooxygenase Activity in Macrophages and Epithelial Cells," *Proc. Natl. Acad. Sci. USA* (October 2000). https://pubmed.ncbi.nlm.nih.gov/11005841/; K. Koba, K. Abe, I. Ikeda, & M. Sugano, "Effects of Alpha-Tocopherol and Tocotrienols on Blood Pressure and Linoleic Acid Metabolism in the Spontaneously Hypertensive Rat (SHR)," *Biosci. Biotechnol. Biochem.* (September 1992); and W. Saksmoto, K. Fujie, J. Nishihira, & M. Mino, "Inhibition of PGE2 Production in Macrophages from Vitamin E-Treated Rats," *Prostaglandins. Leukot. Essent. Fatty Acids* (October 1991). https://pubmed.ncbi.nlm.nih.gov/1745656/

21. I. Simon-Schnass and L. Korniszewski, "The Influence of Vitamin E on Rheological Parameters in High Altitude Mountaineers," *Int. J. Vitam. Nutr. Res.* (1990). https://pubmed.ncbi.nlm.nih.gov/2387667/

22. Michael I. McBurney, Elaine A. Yu, Eric D. Ciappio, Julia K. Bird, et al., "Suboptimal Serum α-Tocopherol Concentrations Observed among Younger Adults and Those Depending Exclusively upon Food Sources," *PLoS One* (August 2015). https://pubmed.ncbi.nlm.nih.gov/26287975/

23. Krisitna E. Hill, Thomas J. Montine, Amy K. Motley, & Xia Le, et al., "Combined Deficiency of Vitamins E and C Causes Paralysis and Death in Guinea Pigs," *Am. J. Clin. Nutr.* (June 2003). https://pubmed.ncbi.nlm.nih.gov/12791628/

24. Y. Koshihara, K. Hoshi, & M. Shiraki, "Vitamin K2 (menatetrenone) inhibits prostaglandin synthesis in cultured human osteoblast-like periosteal cells by inhibiting prostaglandin H synthase activity," *Biochem. Pharmacolo.* (October 1993). https://pubmed.ncbi.nlm. nih.gov/8240383/; and K. Hara, Y. Akiyama, T. Tajima, & M. Shiraki, "Menatetrenone Inhibits Bone Resorption Partly through Inhibition of PGE2 Synthesis in Vitro," *J. Bone Miner. Res.* (May 1993). https://pubmed.ncbi.nlm.nih.gov/8511981/

25. H.M.H. Spronk, B.A.M. Soute, L.J. Schurgers, H.H.W. Thijseen, et al., "Tissue-Specific Utilization of Menaquinone-4 Results in the Prevention of Arterial Calcification in Warfarin-Treated Rats," *J. Vasc. Res.* (November-December 2003). https://pubmed.ncbi.nlm. nih.gov/14654717/; and H. Kawashima, Y. Nakajima, Y. Matubara, J. Nakanowatari, et al., "Effects of Vitamin K2 (menatetrenone) on Atherosclerosis and Blood Coagulation in Hypercholesterolemic Rabbits," *Jpn. J. Pharmacol.* (October 1997). https://pubmed.ncbi. nlm.nih.gov/9414028/

26. M. Otsuka, N. Kato, T. Ichimura, S. Abe, et al., "Vitamin K2 Binds 17beta-hydroxysteroid dehydrogenase 4 and modulates estrogen metabolism," *Life Sci.* (April 2005). https://pubmed.ncbi.nlm.nih. gov/15763078/

27. Wikipedia, "Citric Acid Cycle," last modified January 5, 2022. https://en.wikipedia.org/wiki/Citric_acid_cycle

28. M. Majeed, N. Perskvist, J.D. Ernst, K. Orselius, et al., "Roles of Calcium and Annexins in Phagocytosis and Elimination of an Attenuated Strain of Mycobacterium Tuberculosis in Human Neutrophils," *Microbial Pathogensis*, vol. 24, issue 5 (May 1998). https://www.sciencedirect.com/science/article/abs/pii/S088 240109790200X

29. "High Doses of Calcium May Decrease Severity of E. Coli Symptoms," *Web MD* forum (September 4, 2003); and Ingeborg M.J. Bovee-Oudenhoven, Mischa L. G. Lettink-Wissink, Wim Van Doesburg, Ben J.M. Witteman, et al. "Diarrhea Caused by enterotoxigenic Escherichia Coli Infection of Humans is Inhibited by Dietary Calcium," *Gastroenterology* (August 2003). https:// pubmed.ncbi.nlm.nih.gov/12891550/

30. J.R. Zivin, T. Gooley. R.A. Zager, & M.J. Ryan, "Hypocalcemia: A Pervasive Metabolic Abnormality in the Critically Ill," *Am. J. Kidney Dis.* (April 2001). https://pubmed.ncbi.nlm.nih.gov/11273867/; and D. Aderka, D. Schwartz, M. Dan, & Y. Levo, "Bacteremic Hypocalcemia. A Comparison Between the Calcium Levels of Bacteremic and Nonbacteremic Patients with Infection," *Arch. Intern Med.* (February 1987). https://pubmed.ncbi.nlm.nih.gov/3545115/

31. Majeed, et al., "Roles of Calcium and Annexins in Phagocytosis and Elimination of an Attenuated Strain of Mycobacterium Tuberculosis in Human Neutrophils."

32. American Osteopathic Association, "Low Magnesium Levels Make Vitamin D Ineffective," *sciencedaily.com* (February 2018). https://www.sciencedaily.com/releases/2018/02/180226122548.htm

33. Sara Castiglioni, Alessandra Cazzaniga, Walter Albisetti, & Jeanette A.M. Maiere, "Magnesium and Osteoporosis: Current State of Knowledge and Future Research Directions," *Nutrients* (August 2013). https://www.ncbi.nlm.nih.gov/pmc/articles/PMC3775240/

34. American Osteopathic Association, "Low Magnesium Levels Make Vitamin D Ineffective."

35. Morton Satin, "Salt and our Health," *The Weston A. Price Foundation* (March 2012). https://www.westonaprice.org/health-topics/abcs-of-nutrition/salt-and-our-health/

36. M.H. Alderman, S. Madhavan, H. Cohen, J.E. Sealey, et al., "Low urinary Sodium is Associated with Greater Risk of Myocardial Infarction Among Treated Hypertensive Men," *Hypertension* (June 1995). https://pubmed.ncbi.nlm.nih.gov/7768554/; and M.H. Alderman, H. Cohen, & S. Madhavan, "Dietary Sodium Intake and Mortality," *The Lancet* (March 1998). https://pubmed.ncbi.nlm.nih.gov/9519949/

37. Rajesh Garg, Gordon H. Williams, Shelley Hurwitz, Nancy J. Brown, et al., "Low-Salt Diet Increases Insulin Resistance in Healthy Subjects," *Metabolism* (July 2011). https://pubmed.ncbi.nlm.nih.gov/21036373/

38. Ibid.

39. Ibid.

40. Dr. Jason Fung, "The Salt Scam," drjasonfung.medium.com (September 2018). https://drjasonfung.medium.com/the-salt-scam -1973d73dccd

41. National Institutes of Health, "Selenium: Fact Sheet for Health Professionals," last updated March 26, 2021. https://ods.od.nih. gov/factsheets/Selenium-HealthProfessional/

42. National Institutes of Health, "Zinc: Fact Sheet for Health Professionals," last updated December 2, 2021. https://ods.od.nih. gov/factsheets/Zinc-HealthProfessional/

43. National Institutes of Health, "Copper: Fact Sheet for Health Professionals," last updated March 29, 2021. https://ods.od.nih. gov/factsheets/Copper-HealthProfessional/

## Sleep

1. Centers for Disease Control and Prevention, "Data and Statistics: Short Sleep Duration Among US Adults," last reviewed May 2, 2017. https://www.cdc.gov/sleep/data_statistics.html

2. University of California Berkeley, "Jet-Lagged and Forgetful? It's No Coincidence: Memory, Learning Problems Persist Long After Periods of Jet Lag," *sciencedaily.com* (November 2010). https:// www.sciencedaily.com/releases/2010/11/101124171538.htm; and Matthew Walker, *Why We Sleep: Unlocking the Power of Sleep and Dreams* (Scribner, 2017).

3. Kendra Cherry, "The 4 Stages of Sleep," *Very Well Health* (December 2021). https://www.verywellhealth.com/the-four-stages-of-sleep -2795920# citation-9

4. Joshua E. Brinkman, Vamsi Reddy, & Sandeep Sharma, "Physiology of Sleep," *StatPearls* (September 2021). https://www. ncbi.nlm.nih.gov/books/NBK482512/

5. Bjorn Rasch and Jan Born, "About Sleep's Role in Memory," *Physiol. Rev.* (April 2013). https://pubmed.ncbi.nlm.nih.gov /23589831/; and Danielle Pacheco and Dr. Anis Rehman, "Memory and Sleep," *Sleep Foundation* (November 2020). https:// www.sleepfoundation.org/how-sleep-works/memory-and-sleep

6. Centers for Disease Control and Prevention, "Drowsy Driving," last reviewed March 21, 2017. https://www.cdc.gov/sleep/about_sleep/drowsy_driving.html

7. Rosie Osmun, "Microsleep and the Mind: What's Happening and Why," *Early Bird by Amerisleep* (September 2021). https://amerisleep.com/blog/microsleep/

8. Pacheco and Rehman, "Memory and Sleep."; and Centers for Disease Control and Prevention, "Drowsy Driving."

9. Edward C. Harding, Nicholas P. Franks, & William Wisden, "The Temperature Dependence of Sleep," *Front. Neurosci.* (April 2019). https://www.frontiersin.org/articles/10.3389/fnins.2019.00336/full; and Kazue Okamoto-Mizuno and Koh Mizuno, "Effects of Thermal Environment on Sleep and Circadian Rhythm," *Journal of Physiological Anthropology* (May 2012). https://jphysiolanthropol.biomedcentral.com/articles/10.1186/1880-6805-31-14

## Exercise

1. Brian P. Dunleavy, "One-fifth of US Adults Live with Chronic Pain, Study Estimates," *United Press International* (April 2021). https://www.upi.com/Health_News/2021/04/20/chronic-pain-prevalence-study/9271618927434/

2. Dr. Lin Kooi Ong, "The Tale of High Cortisol Levels, Shrinking Brain and Cognitive Impairment Among Adults in Their 40s," *American Stroke Association* (January 2019). https://journals.heart.org/bloggingstroke/2019/01/22/the-tale-of-high-cortisol-levels-shrinking-brain-and-cognitive-impairment-among-adults-in-their-40s/

## Meditation

1. M. Goyal, S. Singh, E.M.S. Sibinga, N.F. Gould, et al., "Meditation programs for psychological stress and well-being: A Systematic Review and Meta-Analysis," *JAMA Intern. Med.* (March 2014). https://pubmed.ncbi.nlm.nih.gov/24395196/

2. E.H. Kozasa, L.H. Tanaka, C. Monson, S. Little, et al., "The Effects of Meditation-Based Interventions on the Treatment of Fibromyalgia," *Curr. Pain Headache Rep.* (October 2012). https://pubmed.ncbi.nlm.

nih.gov/22717699/; and Ariel J. Lang, Jennifer L. Strauss, Jessica Bomyea, Jill E. Bormann, et al., "The Theoretical and Empirical Basis for Meditation as an Intervention for PTSD," *Behav. Modif.* (November 2012). https://pubmed.ncbi.nlm.nih.gov/22669968/

3. Brigid Schulte, "Harvard Neuroscientist: Meditation Not Only Reduces Stress, Here's How it Changes Your Brain," *The Washington Post* (May 2015). https://www.washingtonpost.com/news/inspired-life/wp/2015/05/26/harvard-neuroscientist-med-itation -not-only-reduces-stress-it-literally-changes-your-brain/

4. Yolanda Lau, "Increasing Mindfulness in the Workplace," *Forbes* (October 2020). https://www.forbes.com/sites/forbeshu-manresourcescouncil/2020/10/05/increasing-mindfulness -in-the-workplace/?sh=4d1d47636956

5. Sara W. Lazar, Catherine E. Kerr, Rachel H. Wasserman, Jeremy R. Gray, et al., "Meditation Experience is Associated with Increased Cortical Thickness," *Neuroreport* (November 2005). https://www.ncbi.nlm.nih.gov/pmc/articles/PMC1361002/; and Britta K. Holzel, James Carmody, Mark Vangel, Christina Congelton, et al., "Mindfulness Practice Leads to Increases in Regional Brain Gray Matter Density," *Psychiatry Res.* (January 2011). https://www.ncbi.nlm.nih.gov/pmc/articles/PMC3004979/

# Illustration Credits

## Chapter 3

Figure 3.1. *Source:* Data from Elizabeth Millard, "How to Balance Your Cortisol Levels," *Experience Life by Life Time* (March 7, 2016). https://experiencelife.lifetime.life/article/the-cortisol-curve/

Figure 3.2. *Source:* Data from Ben Greenfield, "Two Ways Your Brain Breaks and Exactly What You Can Do About It: Part 2," *Ben Greenfield Life - Fitness, Diet, Fat Loss and Performance Advice* (October 22, 2020). https://bengreenfieldlife.com/article/brain-articles/how-to -fix-hpa-axis-dysfunction/

Figure 3.3. *Source:* Data from "Sex-related Symptoms in Men." *Hompes Method.* http://hompes-method.com/hompes-method-for-healthy -menstrual-cycles-and-sex-lives/sex-related-symptoms-in-men/

## Chapter 5

Figure 5.1. Data is credited to Sabelskaya, Getty Images.

## Chapter 12

Figure 12.1. Image is in the public domain, courtesy of USDA Agricultural Research Service.

## Chapter 13

Figure 13.1. *Source:* Data obtained courtesy of the Centers for Disease Control and Prevention.

Figure 13.2. *Source:* Data from Chris Knobbe and Marija Stojanoska, "Diseases of Civilization: Are Seed Oil Excesses the Unifying Mechanism?" (Power Point, Ancestral Health Foundation, Sheraton Denver Downtown Hotel, June 13, 2020).

## Chapter 15

Figure 15.1. *Source:* Data from Chris Knobbe and Marija Stojanoska, "Diseases of Civilization: Are Seed Oil Excesses the Unifying Mechanism?" (Power Point, Ancestral Health Foundation, Sheraton Denver Downtown Hotel, June 13, 2020).

Figure 15.2. *Source:* Carol J Fabian, Bruce F Kimler, and Stephen D Hursting, "Omega-3 Fatty Acids for Breast Cancer Prevention and Survivorship," *PubMed* (May 2015). DOI:10.1186/s1305 -015-0571-6.

# About the Authors

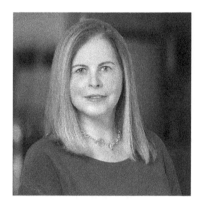

**Dr. Lenae White, MD** was born in Houston, Texas, but spent much of her childhood overseas—in the Caribbean and in the Middle East. Growing up, Lenae had an avid love of horses and was an accomplished equestrian.

Lenae studied chemistry, receiving her undergraduate degree from Texas A & M University. She worked in business for the petrochemical industry for four years before entering medical school in 1992. Lenae went on to Mayo Clinic after medical school to study psychiatry and internal medicine, learning the Mayo way of comprehensive patient care and looking for a way to help patients overcome the scourge of addiction. She was invited to University of Pennsylvania to complete a four-year fellowship in Addiction Psychiatry. This allowed her to work on research and clinical trials with some of the country's pre-eminent clinicians and leaders in addiction treatment and long-term behavioral change. Lenae has continued to be an ardent supporter of advancing the treatment of addiction and continues to work toward reducing the rate of relapse among those recovering. She has been treating addictions successfully for seventeen years.

Throughout her career, Lenae has always had an interest in promoting healing, health, and overall well-being. Recognizing that life creates numerous stressors, she experiences and promotes the value of stress reduction through massage therapy, fitness, diet, and good mental and emotional self-care.

Some time ago, Lenae entered a period of substantial life stressors as did many Americans following the financial crisis of 2008-2009.

Exhausting traditional medical resources trying to "feel better," knowing that something was physiologically wrong, she became frustrated when modern medicine could not identify anything they were able to treat. Various providers suggested that her symptoms would get better when her stress levels were reduced. She came to realize that they were right in one way—that stress was a big part of her problem. But what she came to appreciate, that they had not, was that stress had already been causing damage and was leading her down the road to diseases that would require medical treatment if not addressed. As Lenae explored more natural medicinal remedies for her symptoms, she met Dr. Larry Davis. Working together, they identified many of the underlying root causes of her symptoms and began to work to reverse them. As a result, she did not develop diabetes, entered menopause at a normal age, and did not require any prescribed medications.

Now, seeing the significant impact that co-morbid conditions and obesity were making on mortality and morbidity with COVID-19, Dr. White began to realize that our lifestyle, our food products, and our general dietary choices have been having a very negative impact on the health and wellness of our society. With a passion for helping patients transform and embrace long-lasting behavioral and lifestyle changes to minimize their risks and optimize their overall health and wellness, Dr. White partnered with Dr. Larry Davis to start a wellness company and to write this book, believing that information is power.

Dr. Lenae White splits her time between Texas and Wyoming and enjoys horseback riding and time with her family and two horses.

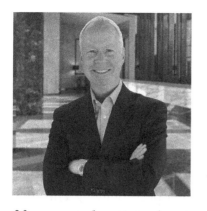

**Dr. Larry Davis, DC** spent much of his childhood in Spokane, Washington. His interest in how the body works and ways to build and improve began in adolescence. He began studying martial arts at the age of twelve and has continued to study many styles throughout his life. As a teen and young adult, he was an accomplished Golden Gloves boxer. Over the last fifteen years he attained an impressive level in the Chinese "internal martial arts" style of Cheng Ming—which includes Tai Chi, Hsing Yi, and Ba Gua—becoming an "in-room" student in 2014.

He attended Kennesaw University in Atlanta, Georgia, for undergraduate education. Because of his lifelong interest in the function and nutrition of the human body, he worked during college as a personal trainer, with certifications from the National Academy of Sports Medicine. After a back injury, Larry was inspired to attend Life West Chiropractic College in Hayward, California, and graduated Summa Cum Laude in 1997. With a doctorate degree under his belt and the influence of Chinese martial arts, he studied and acquired a fellowship from the International Academy of Medical Acupuncture in 2003, further expanding his knowledge of this ancient system and the intricacies of the human body.

In Dallas, Texas, in 2004, Dr. Davis established one of the busiest wellness centers in the country, dedicated to empowering patients to embrace health and vitality throughout all stages of life. He incorporated individualized educational programs designed to remind the body of its origins and to restore and replenish every day. His programs incorporated chiropractic, nutrition, and superior supplements from the earth's "natural pharmacy" and utilized many other supportive modalities, including Medical Hypnotherapy, which he studied intensely in 2006.

However, after being in practice for a short time, Larry himself was diagnosed with hyperthyroidism (high thyroid). Because he was unwilling to accept the "traditional medical model" of treatment for this condition, he researched and used a natural protocol to heal himself. He intensely believes that our bodies possess an innate intelligence with the ability to heal and restore themselves when given the right environment. He thus has focused the entirety of his post-graduate education on the study of hormonal and nutritional physiology, assisting patients to reach their full potential. Dr. Davis is that new breed of doctor who practices what he preaches.

His concurrent interest in the mind-body connection led to years of study in meditation and spirituality in the quest for equanimity. Dr. Davis has been meditating daily for almost three decades. He considers this practice one of the most important aspects of living a healthy and centered life. He is taking his vision of health and wellness into the business world, partnering with Dr. Lenae White to incorporate optimal wellness and peak performance into the corporate culture.

Dr. Davis resides in Dallas, Texas, with his best friend and spousal equivalent of twenty years. He is an avid reader and enjoys nothing more than spending time with her and their rescued dogs, Khana and Crosby.